Pharmacology, Doping and Sports

The work of dope testers is constantly being obstructed by the development of ever harder-to-trace new forms of banned substances. Organisations such as the World Anti-Doping Association and the United States Anti-Doping Agency are pioneering cutting-edge techniques designed to keep competition at the highest level fair and safe, and must ensure that their drug-testing laboratories adhere to the highest scientific standards. In *Pharmacology, Doping and Sports*, these techniques and procedures are explained by the anti-doping experts who practice them.

Broad-ranging in scope, this book examines the effects of performance-enhancing substances on the athlete's health and the role of anti-doping procedures as an ethical question. Additionally, it explains the background to, and the emergence of, the anti-doping movement. The book also offers in-depth analysis of key scientific matters, such as:

- standard analytical and diagnostic tests for sports doping
- regulatory standards for laboratory proficiency
- common performance-enhancing techniques such as anabolic and designer steroids, blood doping, growth hormones, and gene doping
- carbon isotope ratio testing

Written by some of the world's leading authorities on the science of sports doping, *Pharmacology, Doping and Sports* provides an invaluable study of up-to-the-minute anti-doping techniques. This book is essential reading for all sports scientists, coaches, policy-makers, students and athletes interested in the science or ethics of doping in sport.

Jean L Fourcroy is a regulatory consultant in urology and endocrinology, and a leading authority on the science of anti-doping. She has been appointed to the Board of the United States Anti-Doping Agency, is an active member of the American Urological Association and the American Society of Andrology, and is a Past President of the American Medical Women's Association.

Pharmacology, Doping and Sports

A scientific guide for athletes, coaches, physicians, scientists and administrators

Edited by Jean L Fourcroy

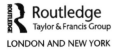
Routledge
Taylor & Francis Group

LONDON AND NEW YORK

First published 2009
by Routledge
2 Park Square, Milton Park, Abingdon, Oxon OX14 4RN

Simultaneously published in the USA and Canada
by Routledge
711 Third Avenue, New York, NY 10017

Routledge is an imprint of the Taylor & Francis Group, an informa business

© 2009 Jean L Fourcroy, selection and editorial matter;
individual chapters, the contributors

Typeset in Times New Roman by
Keystroke, 28 High Street, Tettenhall, Wolverhampton

British Library Cataloguing in Publication Data
A catalogue record for this book is available from the British Library

Library of Congress Cataloging-in-Publication Data
Pharmacology, doping and sports: a scientific guide for athletes, coaches,
physicians, scientists and administrators / edited by
Jean L. Fourcroy.
  p.; cm.
Includes bibliographical references.
1. Doping in sports. I. Fourcroy, Jean L.
[DNLM: 1. Doping in Sports—methods. 2. Anabolic
Agents—adverse effects. 3. Doping in Sports—ethics.
4. Steroids—adverse effects. 5. Substance Abuse Detection—methods. QT
261 P536 2008]
RC1230.P53 2008
362.29–dc22   2008011128

ISBN10: 0–415–42845–9 (hbk)
ISBN10: 0–203–89104–X (ebk)

ISBN13: 978–0–415–42845–3 (hbk)
ISBN13: 978–0–203–89104–9 (ebk)

Contents

Notes on contributors

Dr Rodrigo Aguilera completed his B.Sc. M.S. at the university of Lyon and Ph.D. at the CNRS Mass Spectrometry Laboratory in the Chemistry and Biology department. At the CNRS he worked for 5 years to develop a new approach to the detection of performance-enhancing drugs used by professional athletes by measuring the Carbon Isotope Ratio Mass Spectrometry (IRMS). He was then employed at the Olympic Analytical Laboratory headed by Dr Don Catlin in the Department of Medical and Molecular Pharmacology at UCLA where he worked for 4 years. Using the IRMS detection method he developed while in France, Dr Aguilera became an authority in this field, and was one of the pioneers in the application of IRMS to identify the use of exogenous testosterone. He was responsible for the drug testing analysis by IRMS at the Atlanta Summer Olympics, Salt Lake City Winter Olympics and the 2007 Pan American Games as well as at other sporting events. Since joining the Mass Spectrometry Laboratory at UCLA in 2002 Dr Aguilera expanded his experience to the field of proteomics. Dr Aguilera has worked closely with Dr Julian Whitelegge on a US Department of Energy funded project investigating the proteomics of a blue-green alga. In 2003 Dr Aguilera helped to establish and directed the University of Southern California Proteomics Core Facility Laboratory. Since 2006 Dr Aguilera has established and directed the Proteomics Core Facility at the House Ear Institute.

Christiane Ayotte has been Director of the Doping Control Laboratory, INRS – Institut Armand-Frappier, Quebec, since 1991. She has been a member of the IAAF Doping Commission since 1995 and of the IOC Working Group on Harmonization of Laboratory Protocols since 1996, and was elected representative of the Heads of IOC Accredited Laboratories in 1995–6.

Larry D Bowers serves on the WADA Laboratory Accreditation Subcommittee. He served as Deputy Director of the drug-testing laboratory for the 1996 Olympic Games in Atlanta and 1999 Pan Am Games in Canada. He also received the MCF LS Palmer Award for outstanding contributions to chromatography in 1985, and the annual Franklin &

Marshall College Alumni Citation in 2007 for distinguished professional contributions.

Richard V Clark is a Clinical Researcher in Endocrinology and Metabolism, and a Group Director in Metabolic Discovery Medicine and Clinical Pharmacology at GlaxoSmithKline. Prior to moving to GSK, Dr Clark was in academic medicine, initially on faculty at Emory University School of Medicine, Atlanta, and then at Duke University Medical Center, Durham. He is a past president of the American Society of Andrology.

Jean L Fourcroy is a regulatory consultant in urology and endocrinology, and a leading authority on the science of anti-doping. She has been appointed to the Board of USADA and is an active member of the American Urological Association and the American Society of Andrology, and past president of the American Medical Women's Association.

Theodore Friedmann is Professor of Pediatrics at the Center for Molecular Genetics, School of Medicine, University of California, San Diego. The primary area of research for his laboratory is gene therapy. Professor Friedmann was named president of the American Society of Gene Therapy in 2006. He is also Director of the interdepartmental UCSD Gene Therapy Program and Whitehill Chair of Biomedical Ethics.

Richard L Hilderbrand joined USADA in March 2003 as Science Director, where he currently manages the Therapeutic Use Exemption process. He is retired from the Navy, where his last assignment was at the Office of the Secretary of Defense, The Pentagon, where he had primary responsibility for drug abuse reduction programs for the military services.

Richard Holt became Reader in Endocrinology and Metabolism at the University of Southampton in 2006. His current research interests are broadly focused around the GH–IGF axis and the pathogenesis of the insulin resistance syndrome. These studies have led on to research into the development of a test for the detection of GH abuse in sport. He has acted as an adviser to WADA and USADA.

Françoise Lasne is head of the Research and Biological Development Department at the French National Anti-Doping Laboratory. Dr Lasne developed the first urine test for detection of recombinant human erythropoietin (EPO) in 1999. This form of testing, first used in Sydney at the 2000 Olympic Games, is now used by all international anti-doping agencies.

Stephen Muza is a research physiologist at the US Army Research Institute of Environmental Medicine in Natick, MA. Dr Muza has investigated high-altitude sickness, physiological adaptations to high altitude, human performance at high altitude and control of respiration. He has authored over 100 peer-reviewed articles in scholarly journals, and many textbook chapters.

Andrew Pipe is the Director of the Minto Prevention and Rehabilitation Centre at the University of Ottawa Heart Institute. He is also a Professor at the Faculty of Medicine, University of Ottawa, Ontario, Canada. He was the founding Chair of Physicians for a Smoke-Free Canada and was made an honorary life member of the Canadian Council on Smoking and Health in 1989. In addition, he is Team Physician for the Canadian National Men's Basketball Team and Chair Emeritus of the Canadian Centre for Ethics and Sport.

Baaron Pittinger joined the United States Olympic Committee (USOC) in 1977 as Director of Special Events. He subsequently served the USOC as Assistant Executive Director (1981–7) and Executive Director (1988–90) prior to being named Executive Director of US Hockey (1990–3). Pittinger was awarded the prestigious Olympic Order by the International Olympic Committee in 1992.

Michael N Sawka is Chief of the Thermal and Mountain Medicine Division at the U.S. Army Research Institute of Environmental Medicine in Natick, MA. His research interests are environmental and exercise physiology, fluid/electrolyte balance and rehabilitation medicine. He has authored over 200 peer-reviewed articles in scholarly journals, and many textbook chapters.

Peter H Sönksen is Emeritus Professor of Endocrinology at St Thomas' Hospital and King's College London, and Visiting Professor at Southampton University Medical School. Professor Sönksen's group were the first to discover the syndrome of "growth hormone deficiency in adults" (1991) and to demonstrate the benefits of growth hormone replacement (1989). He has worked for the IOC Medical Commission as an expert on growth hormones.

Carl Swenson has been a USADA Board Member since 2007, and is attending the University of Utah S.J. Quinney School of Law. He represented the United States both in mountain biking and in cross-country skiing, appearing as a representative in the latter at the 1994, 2002 and 2006 Olympic Winter Games.

Travis T Tygart is the Chief Executive Officer of the United States Anti-Doping Agency (USADA). As part of his duties, he investigated the BALCO doping conspiracy, and arbitrated over 30 cases before the AAA or CAS, including the cases of Tim Montgomery, Michelle Collins and Chryste Gaines. He was involved with drafting the USADA Protocol for Olympic Movement Testing and the World Anti-Doping Agency's Code.

Andrew J Young is a research physiologist and Chief of the Military Nutrition Division at the US Army Research Institute of Environmental Medicine in Natick, MA. Dr Young has investigated the biological basis for, and strategies to mitigate, performance degradations in people exposed to stressors such as intense physical exertion, nutritional deprivation and exposure to extremes of heat, cold and high altitude.

Foreword

On behalf of the USADA Board of Directors, staff and the thousands of clean athletes that USADA represents, it is my pleasure and privilege to write a foreword for this important book. Many people consider doping to be the biggest danger facing players and sport today. From the player's perspective, the use of performance-enhancing drugs creates an atmosphere of coercion where clean athletes, who do not want to take drugs, feel compelled to do so in order to succeed. In the age of fame and multimillion-dollar rewards for athletic success, the siren call of drugs has become even more alluring.

While some claim that doping is a victimless violation of the rules, the true victims of doping are the athletes who wish to complete clean and are denied this opportunity. Essentially, every athlete's right to play clean is violated when one athlete decides to cheat by using drugs. Additionally, the sport itself and the public are harmed by being defrauded when athletic performances are ruined through the use of drugs. How sad it is when one of our heroes is exposed as nothing more than a sports fraud. Similarly, doping compromises our fundamental values since doping represents the loss of ethics and integrity that comes from cheating.

Sport, with its focus on healthy competition, culture and fundamental human values, affects our lives probably more than any other event, athletic or otherwise. Participation in sport, as an athlete or fan, fosters relationships with others that transcend race, religion, gender and economic disparities while simultaneously developing healthy participants. All of these benefits of athletic competition lead to great personal and societal accomplishment.

Like many of you with children, I get a thrill watching my 6-year-old daughter struggle through a soccer match and attempt to overcome the obstacles in her way, not because I truly believe she will be the next Mia Hamm but because I know that the lessons she learns on the playing field will remain a powerful repository of strength and self-confidence at every stage and area of her life.

It makes perfectly good sense why, teenage pregnancy is lower for girls who play sports, and why women who play sports are 60 percent less likely to get breast cancer, and have higher levels of self-esteem and suffer less from depression and obesity.

Hopefully, this casebook will further educate its readers on the importance of ethical competition and, just like sport played by the rules, will foster the growth of the values we all still cherish.

Travis T Tygart
Chief Executive Officer
USADA

Preface

Is this an Olympic chemical race or a race to the swift of the enhanced?

I seem to have spent the greater part of my life looking at the science of "doping" as a urologist, a regulatory scientist and an anabolic steroid expert at the Food and Drug Administration and now as a member of the Board of the United States Anti-Doping Agency. During these years, I have had the opportunity to learn first-hand about the abuse of drugs and use of methods. It has been an honor to work with the Drug Enforcement Agency to bring about change, and to be an expert in such cases as the Dan Duchane case.

During these years, we have come from the dietary supplement of choice – andostenedione – to the development of sophisticated agents such as erythopoietin (EPO), which unfortunately probably killed many through the overproduction of red blood cells. With the development of new drugs came the development of new laboratory instrumentation and expertise. The validation and accreditation of our laboratories requires the best and it is a pleasure to share with you the best of science today. These are the world's experts who work to keep our athletes clean.

We are all dedicated to preserving the well-being of Olympic sport and integrity of competition while ensuring the health of athletes.

Jean L Fourcroy

Prologue
An athlete's perspective

In my 13 years of mountain bike and cross-country ski racing, not one season passed without news of a fellow competitor being banned for using a performance-enhancing drug. With every cheater caught, rumors and suspicion surrounded numerous others. At several major events, doping scandals outplayed the athletics; clean athletes were tainted and discouraged, fans were disillusioned, and many sponsors left these small market sports entirely. The elimination of widespread cynicism prevalent in many sports will require aggressive anti-doping tactics on several fronts. One bright spot in the fight against doping is the advances in scientific research and drug testing. Leading the way, and a model for the rest of the world, is the approach taken by the United States Anti-Doping Agency (USADA).

USADA, independent from any single sports federation, has the resources to develop up-to-date drug tests and the power to execute effective doping controls. All elite athletes competing in Olympic sports are required to submit their whereabouts to USADA at all times. Any active athlete can expect a USADA doping control officer to show up at his or her door at any time of the year requesting a urine sample (soon a blood sample will also be on the menu). While these measures compromise privacy and convenience, a clean athlete gains a more level playing field, and the athlete tempted to cheat is given more incentive to stay clean.

Unfortunately, the lure that a banned drug provides to some athletes will never disappear. New drugs and new techniques will always be a temptation to those who think they can beat the doping controls. Constant research and new tests are crucial to keep the cheaters in check, or, at the very least, increase the risk and costs of attempting to evade detection. Every profession has its cheaters. The more lucrative and competitive a business is, the greater the incentive to gain an advantage by going outside the rules. Once the perception of widespread cheating is established, true or not, it becomes easier for previously honest athletes to rationalize cheating. High-level sports have arrived at this level of corruption. Scientific research and sophisticated testing systems are the most effective tools in helping to rebalance the playing field.

As an athlete, I was grateful for the efforts of the Anti-Doping Agencies and willing to accept the anti-doping protocols in exchange for the leveling effect they brought to my sports. As a retired athlete and fan of sports in general, I recognize the broader value of promoting clean sports, and support anti-doping agencies in their efforts keep the science on pace with that of the dopers.

Carl Swenson

Acknowledgments

This book is only possible due to the commitment by the United States Anti-Doping Agency (USADA) on scientific research. Additionally, without the support of dedicated scientists and clean athletes, this book could not have happened. Special thanks goes to our dedicated accredited laboratories around the world. Special thanks to Dr Larry Bowers, USADA's Senior Managing Director, and the entire dedicated staff and Board of USADA. We all support the athletes' statement: My Health, My Sport, My Victory.

Abbreviations

AAA	American Arbitration Association
AAS	anabolic-androgenic steroids
AAV	adeno-associated recombinant virus
ADD	attention deficit disorder
ADHD	attention deficit hyperactivity disorder
AGAL	Australian Government Analytical Laboratories
ALS	acid-labile subunit
AOA	(former) American Olympic Association
BRP	Biological Reference Preparation
C	combustion
CAM	crassulacean acid metabolism
CAS	Court of Arbitration for Sport
CASPER	Coalition for Anabolic Steroid Precursor and Ephedra Regulation
CAWIA	Commission on Atomic Weights and Isotopic Abundances
CCD	charge-coupled device
cDNA	complementary DNA
CERA	Continuous Erythropoiesis Receptor Activator
CHO	Chinese hamster ovary
CIR	carbon isotope ratio
DB	double blotting
DHEA	dehydroepiandrosterone
DHT	dihydrotestosterone
DMT	desoxymethyltestosterone
EI	electronic impact
EIA	exercise-induced asthma
EIB	exercise-induced bronchospasm
ELISA	enzyme-linked immunosorbent assay
EPO	erythropoietin
ERC	endogenous reference compound
ESI	electrospray ionization
EU	European Union

FDA	Food and Drug Administration (United States)
FID	flame ionization detector
FIFA	Fédération Internationale de Football Association
FIS	Fédération Internationale de Ski (International Ski Federation)
GC	gas chromatograph/gas chromatography
GH	growth hormone
GHDA	growth hormone deficiency in adults
GHRH	growth-hormone-releasing hormone
hCG	human chorionic gonadotrophin
Hct	hematocrit
HDL	high-density lipoprotein
hGH	human growth hormone
HPLC	high-performance liquid chromatography
IAAF	International Amateur Athletics Federation
IAEA	International Atomic Energy Agency
ICAS	International Council of Arbitration for Sport
ICTP	C-terminal cross-linked telopeptide of Type 1 collagen
IEF	isoelectric focusing
IFs	International Olympic Sports Federations
IGFBP	insulin-like growth factor-binding protein
IGF-I	insulin-like growth factor I
IgG	immunoglobulin G
ILAC	International Laboratory Accreditation Corporation
IM	intramuscular(ly)
IND	investigational new drug application
IOC	International Olympic Committee
IRMS	(carbon) isotope ratio mass spectrometry
ISL	International Standard for Laboratories
IST	International Standard for Testing
IUPAC	International Union of Pure and Applied Chemistry
LBM	lean body mass
LDL	low-density lipoprotein
LH	luteinizing hormone
MDMA	3,4-methylenedioxy-N-methylamphetamine
mRNA	messenger ribonucleic acid
MS	mass spectrometer/mass spectrometry
MWCO	molecular weight cutoff
NESP	Novel Erythropoiesis-Stimulating Protein
NGB	National Governing Body
NIDA	National Institute on Drug Abuse (United States)
NIH	National Institutes of Health (United States)
NOC	National Olympic Committee
OBA	Office of Biotechnology Activities (United States)
OCOGs	Organizing Committees of the Olympic Games

OHRP	Office of Human Research Protection (United States)
OMADC	Olympic Movement Anti-Doping Code
PDB	Pee Dee Belemnite
PEG	polyethylene glycol
PICP	C-terminal propeptide of Type 1 collagen
P-III-P	procollagen Type 3 N-terminal peptide
PVDF	polyvinylidene fluoride
RAC	Recombinant DNA Advisory Committee (United States)
rEPO	recombinant erythropoietin
Ret Hct	reticulocyte hematocrit
rhEPO	recombinant erythropoietin
rhGH	recombinant human growth hormone
SCID	severe combined immunodeficiency diseases
SELDI-TOF MS	surface-enhanced laser desorption/ionization time-of-flight mass spectrometry
SIM	selective ion monitoring
SPE	solid-phase extraction
sTfr	soluble receptors of transferrin
T/E	testosterone to epitestosterone ratio
THE	tetrahydrocortisone
THF	tetrahydrocortisol
THG	tetrahydrogestrinone
TMS	trimethylsilyl
TUE	therapeutic use exemption
UCI	Union Cycliste Internationale
UNESCO	United Nations Educational, Scientific and Cultural Organization
USADA	United States Anti-Doping Agency
USOA	(former) United States Olympic Association
USOC	United States Olympic Committee
VPDB	Vienna Pee Dee Belemnite
WAADS	World Association of Anti-Doping Scientists
WADA	World Anti-Doping Agency

1   The historical and scientific pathway to fair and accurate testing

Jean L Fourcroy and Baaron Pittinger

1 Introduction

> The most important thing in the Olympic Games is not to win but to take part, just as the most important thing in life is not the triumph but the struggle. The essential thing is not to have conquered but to have fought well.
>
> (The Olympic Creed[1])

> In the name of all competitors, I promise that we shall take part in these Olympic Games, respecting and abiding by the rules which govern them, in the true spirit of sportsmanship, for the glory of sport and the honor of our teams.
>
> (The Olympic Oath, delivered by an athlete of the host nation during the Opening Ceremonies[2])

Given these two foundations on which athlete participation in the Games rests, it is obvious why the battle against doping in sport is of such importance to the Olympic Movement. Further, among the stated objectives of the International Olympic Committee is the promotion of the Olympics throughout the world by encouraging and supporting ethics in sport, and dedicating its efforts to ensuring that in sport, the spirit of fair play prevails. Simply put, doping is antithetical to the spirit of the Games. In recent years doping scandals have tarnished the Games, but the International Olympic Committee (IOC) and other responsible members of the Olympic family are making a determined effort to restore their integrity.

2 The beginnings

The Olympic Games have a long history. Olympic sport was first recorded in 776 BC, but may have begun as early as the thirteenth century BC. The Greeks based their chronology on four-year periods called Olympiads (a practice that has been retained in the modern games), dating from 776 BC, and the Olympic festival marked the beginning of each Olympiad. The festival was a religious event to celebrate the gods, but primarily Zeus, worshiped in common by all Hellenes. There were three other major pan-Hellenic festivals, all of which included fairs, but the festival at Olympia had become pre-eminent by 572 BC, when Elis and Sparta entered into an alliance under which Elis was in charge of the event itself, while Sparta enforced the sacred 30-day no-war truce.[3]

A single foot race the length of the stadium, approximately 200 yards, was the only athletic event until the fifteenth Olympiad, when other types of sports began to make their way into the festival: wrestling and the pentathlon in 708 BC, boxing in 688 BC, and chariot racing in 680 BC. At one time or another, there were 23 Olympic sports events, but they were never all conducted at the same festival.

A wild olive branch was the only official prize for an Olympic winner, although some unofficial prizes were awarded by city-states. Athens allowed an Olympic champion to live free of charge in the Prytaneum, at a special hall for distinguished citizens. Other city-states exempted winners from taxes for an Olympiad, and in some cases citizens contributed to a cash award. In AD 349, the Roman emperor Theodosius the Great, a devout Christian, decreed an end to the Olympic Games and their celebration of the Greek gods. They had lasted more than a thousand years, and left an ember that burst into flame again in the late nineteenth century.

3 The modern games

Baron de Coubertin is given credit for reestablishing the Games. However, through the years there were more than 40 different events that played off the Olympic theme – frequently in connection with industrial fairs during the industrial revolution.[4,5] It is believed that de Coubertin witnessed earlier Olympic festival games at Chelsea Stadium in London: amateur athletes only, and medals rather than cash prizes. As the line between amateur and profes-sional athletes became increasingly blurred, particularly with the advent of state-sponsored athletes, several international federations have voted to make professionals eligible for participation, with IOC approval.

Baron de Coubertin, who was French, had grown up in the shadow of his country's devastating defeat in the Franco-Prussian War of 1870–1 and was determined to devote his life to education, and especially to physical education. In 1889, he organized the Congress of Physical Education in Paris, and in 1892 he began espousing the idea of a rebirth of the Olympic Games, but attracted little notice. Despite repeated rebuffs, not only from his own countrymen but from the British and Americans as well, de Coubertin persisted. On June 23, 1894, he presided over a meeting of 79 delegates representing 12 countries, who unanimously voted for the restoration of the Olympic Games.[5]

As a result, the IOC was organized in 1894 in Paris with the goal of staging the first modern Olympics in Paris in 1900.[6] Pressed by de Coubertin, the IOC soon decided to aim for 1896, with Athens as the site. That idea, too, met with resistance, especially from the government of Greece. But when Georgios

Averoff of Alexandria donated 920,000 gold drachmas to build an Olympic stadium in Athens, the resistance folded, and the king of Greece himself opened the first modern Olympic Games in 1896.

To the traditional track and field events, which include the marathon and decathlon, a host of sports have been added so that today there are multiple sports on the program of the Summer Games. The Games were strictly for men until 1900 at the Paris Summer Games, when women first took part.[7] The IOC has since significantly increased the participation of women. A separate series of Winter Olympic meets was inaugurated in 1924 at Chamonix, France. The Winter Games are much smaller, are limited to sports that can be contested on either ice or snow, and have begun to include nontraditional sports as the IOC attempts to maintain the Games' appeal to a young audience. After the 1992 Games, the IOC placed the Winter Games on a new cycle, beginning in 1994, with the Summer Games keeping to the same schedule and celebrating the centennial event in Atlanta in 1996.[8]

4 The International Olympic Committee

Today, organizations included in the Olympic Movement are headed by the IOC, the International Federations (IFs), the National Olympic Committees (NOCs), the National Governing Bodies (NGBs) for each sport, which operate under the aegis of the NOCs, and the Organizing Committees of the Olympic Games (OCOGs), which disappear after they have conducted the Games. The IOC, also called the Comité International Olympique, is based in Lausanne, Switzerland; its membership currently includes 206 NOCs. The IOC serves as the umbrella organization and owns all rights to the Olympic symbols, flag, motto, anthem and the Olympic Games themselves. It awards the sites and oversees the organization of the Games by the OCOGs. In addition, the IOC seeks, through a variety of programs, to encourage and support initiatives blending sport with culture and education.[6]

5 The United States Olympic Committee (USOC)

The USOC began as a small group headed by James E. Sullivan, the founder of the Amateur Athletic Union, which entered the 12 US athletes who partic-ipated in the inaugural Olympic Games in Athens in 1896. The delegation was headed by Dr William Milligan Sloane, a Princeton Professor, and all of the athletes had either Princeton or Harvard ties. Sloane served as first president of the committee, and became a close confidant of de Coubertin. The com-mittee was finally formalized as the American Olympic Association (AOA) at a meeting in November 1921 at the New York Athletic Club.[8]

In 1940, the AOA changed its name to the United States of America Sports Federation, and in 1945 changed it again to the United States Olympic Association (USOA). Public Law 805, which granted the USOA a federal charter, was enacted in 1950 and enabled the USOA to solicit tax-deductible contributions as a private, nonprofit corporation. When the USOA made major constitutional revisions in 1961, it adopted its current name, the United States Olympic Committee (USOC). The USOC moved its headquarters from New York City to Colorado Springs on July 1, 1978.[9]

The passage of Public Law 95–606, the Amateur Sports Act (now known as the Ted Stevens Olympic and Amateur Sports Act), on November 8, 1978 was without question the most significant development in the history of the USOC.[10] It specifically named the USOC as the coordinating body for athletic activity in the United States directly relating to international family athletic competition, including the sports on the programs of the Olympic, Paralympic and Pan-American games, strengthened its fund-raising abilities by providing it with exclusive control of Olympic symbols and terminology in the United States, and established each National Governing Body as an independent entity. Prior to passage of the Act, the USOC had been little more than a travel agency concerned with assembling teams for the Olympic and Pan-American Games, outfitting them, and underwriting their travel. The Act, together with changes the USOC made in its own constitution, dramatically affected its role and efficiency. From quadrennial budgets of several million dollars in the 1960s, the USOC has blossomed into an organization that now has four-year budgets in the neighborhood of $500,000, and effectively supports the programs of the various NGBs and the needs of their Olympic team candidates.

From 1969 until early 1985, Colonel F Don Miller served as executive director. He was an exceptional leader and deserves a lion's share of the credit for the changes that occurred during his term. When the IOC asked each National Olympic Committee to name its outstanding individual of the twentieth century, the USOC voted that honor to Colonel Miller. Apart from the progress the USOC achieved on his watch, he guided the organization through one of its most difficult periods. In January 1980, the Carter administration severely pressured the USOC to boycott that summer's Olympic Games in Moscow because of the Soviet invasion of Afghanistan. When a badly torn USOC finally capitulated, its income from corporate sponsorships and public contributions had nearly dried up, but Colonel Miller was able to keep the organization alive.

6 Tarnish on the gold

The Olympic Games have been prey to many factors that have tended to thwart their ideals of world cooperation and athletic excellence. Although officially only individuals win Olympic medals, nations routinely assign political significance to the feats of their citizens and teams, and national medal counts have become a fixture both in the press and by NOCs. That fact was most certainly behind the state-sponsored doping program instituted by East Germany,[11] and perhaps the Soviet Union, during the 1970s and 1980s, which led to a quick spread of doping to individual athletes in a broad range of sports and countries, both within the Games and in other competitions as well.[12] The IOC began a drug testing program at the 1968 Games in Mexico City under the direction of its own Medical Commission, and had only a single positive – for marijuana.

The first major drug scandal from the Games (setting aside the belated discovery of GDR's program) occurred in 1988 when Canadian sprinter Ben Johnson tested positive for anabolic steroid use. The specter of drug cheats has haunted the Games and other major athletic competitions ever since.

7 Turning the tide – the World Anti-Doping Agency and the United States Anti-Doping Agency

Once the doping problem had been identified in the 1980s, a number of national anti-doping agencies were created, but there was no strong leadership from the IOC, and the efforts of the individual agencies was largely fragmented. It took a major scandal surrounding the 1998 Tour de France to finally launch a determined, coordinated worldwide effort to eliminate, or at least curtail, doping. The IOC decided to convene a world conference on doping, bringing together all stakeholders, which was conducted in Lausanne on February 2–4, 1999. The conference produced the Lausanne Declaration on Doping in Sport, which provided for the creation of an independent international anti-doping agency to be fully operational for the Games of the XXVII Olympiad in Sydney, Australia, in 2000. Thus was born the World Anti-Doping Agency (WADA) to promote and coordinate the fight against doping internationally. WADA was established as a foundation under the initiative of the IOC with the support and participation of intergovernmental organizations, governments, public authorities, and other public and private bodies involved with the problem of doping in sport. The agency's board consists of equal representatives from the Olympic Movement and public authorities.

At the same time as the IOC was establishing an independent agency, so was the USOC, and at the conclusion of the Sydney Games the United States Anti-Doping Agency (USADA) opened its doors on October 2, 2000 as the independent anti-doping agency for Olympic-related sport in the United States. The USOC had conducted its own anti-doping program since 1983 and was aware that it was viewed internationally as the fox guarding the hen house. Within the Olympic family, American athletes were considered to be among the very worst of dopers. In June 1999, president Bill Hybl appointed a Select Task Force on Externalization, charged with recommending both the governing structure (as represented by the board of directors) and the responsibilities that would be assumed by the new agency. USADA was given full authority to create and execute a comprehensive anti-doping program encompassing testing, adjudication, education, and research.

Within a period of a few years, USADA emerged as an international leader in the anti-doping battle, and a model for other anti-doping agencies under the direction of its CEO, Terry Madden.

8 The Prohibited List, Laboratory Working Committee, and the Court for Arbitration for Sport

Among the keys to an effective anti-doping program are the legal definition of doping, the Prohibited List, efficient laboratory analysis, and a fair adjudication process. The first Prohibited List, compiled by the IOC Medical Commission, was published in 1963, and the list has been periodically revised ever since. Since 2004, as mandated by WADA's World Anti-Doping Code, WADA is responsible for the preparation and publication of the List. The list is a cornerstone of the Code and a key component of harmonization. It is an international standard identifying substances and methods prohibited in competition, out of competition, and in particular sports. It is published by October 1 and goes into effect on January 1 of the following year.[13]

The WADA Laboratory Working Committee is responsible for providing expert advice, recommendations and guidance to WADA with respect to the overall management of the anti-doping laboratory accreditation and reaccreditation process, for which WADA is responsible.[14] It is also responsible for the maintenance of the International Standard for Laboratories and associated Technical Documents.[14] The science of testing is highly sensitive and specific. At the time of publication, there were 34 WADA-accredited laboratories around the world. Accuracy is necessary to protect and encourage clean athletes.

In 1981, soon after his election as IOC president, His Excellency Juan Antonio Samaranch had the idea of creating a sports-specific jurisdiction. The following year at the IOC Session held in Rome, IOC member His Excellency Kéba Mbaye, who was then a judge at the International Court of Justice in The Hague, chaired a working group tasked with preparing the statutes of what would quickly become the "Court of Arbitration for Sport".[15]

The preamble of the agreement states that

> with the aim of facilitating the resolution of disputes in the world of sport, an arbitration institution entitled "the Court of Arbitration for Sport" (hereinafter the CAS) has been created, and that, with the aim of ensuring the protection of the rights of the parties before the CAS and the absolute independence of this institution, the parties have decided by mutual agreement to create a Foundation for international sports-related arbitration called the "International Council of Arbitration for Sport" (hereinafter the ICAS) under the aegis of which the CAS will henceforth be placed.

9 Summary

The history of doping and the necessity for externalization of doping control, education, and research was apparent by the end of the twentieth century. During the past 50 years, important scientific and technical advances have challenged scientists and provided new performance enhancement tools.

Scientists have had a constant challenge to keep pace with the dopers. The following chapters exemplify this challenge.

Should we perhaps go back to the olive branch?

10 Acknowledgment

We are very grateful for the tremendous history that Baaron Pittinger brings to this chapter.

11 References

1 The Olympic Creed. http://www.usantidoping.org/misc/clean_sport.aspx (accessed December 14, 2007).

2 The Olympic Oath. http://www.olympic.org/uk/index_uk.asp (accessed December 14, 2007).

3 *The Olympic Games in early Greece.* http://users.otenet.gr/~tzelepisk/yc/olymp.htm, http://www.usoc.org/12690.htm (accessed December 14, 2007).

4 Dimeo P. *History of drug use in sport, 1876–1976: beyond good and evil.* London: Routledge, 2007.

5 Pierre de Coubertin, founding father of the modern Olympic Games and the Olympic Movement. Available from http://www.olympic.org/uk/passion/museum/permanent/index_uk.asp (accessed December 14, 2007).

6 The history and formation of the International Olympic Committee. Available from http://www.olympic.org/uk/organisation/ioc/index_uk.asp (accessed December 14, 2007).

7 Modern Olympic Games. Available from http://gtresearchnews.gatech.edu/reshor/rh-win96/timeline.htm (accessed May 23, 2008).

8 The Olympic Movement. Available from http://www.olympic.org/uk/organisation/movement/index_uk.asp (accessed December 14, 2007).

9 Formation of the United States Olympic Committee. Available from www.usocpressbox.org/mediaguide/USOC/usoc_about.doc (accessed December 14, 2007).

10 United States Amateur Sports Act. http://www.whitewaterslalom.org/rules/asa-1978.html (accessed December 14, 2007).

11 Franke WW, Berendonk B. Hormonal doping and androgenization of athletes: a secret program of the German Democratic Republic government. *Clinical Chemistry.* 1997; 43(7): 1262–79.

12 Litsky F. Use of steroids: discovery in the face of disbelief. Available from http://query.nytimes.com/gst/fullpage.html?res=9405E7D61438F93BA1575BC0A965948260&sec=health&spon=&pagewanted=all.

13 The Prohibited List. Available from http://www.wada-ama.org/en/prohibitedlist.ch2 (accessed December 14, 2007).

14 World Anti-Doping Accreditated Laboratories. Available from http://www.wada-ama.org/en/dynamic.ch2?pageCategory.id=333 (accessed December 14, 2007).

15 The Court of Arbitration for Sport. Available from http://www.tas-cas.org/en/info/frminf.htm (accessed December 14, 2007).

2 Ensuring quality results in a global testing system

Larry D Bowers

1 Introduction

Recognition of the problem of performance-enhancing drugs in sport occurred in the 1920s, when the International Amateur Athletics Federation (IAAF) banned the use of stimulants, but without the availability of a test to detect their use. The Union Cycliste Internationale (UCI) and the Fédération Internationale de Football Association (FIFA; soccer) were among the first international sports federations to introduce doping tests in their respective World Championships in the 1960s. The International Olympic Committee (IOC) formed a Medical Commission in 1967 to deal with the perceived increase in drugs and other performance-enhancing substances that not only affected the evenness of the playing field but also exposed the athlete to health risks. In 1982, the IOC came to an agreement with the IAAF, whose medical commission had established standards for accrediting anti-doping laboratories, to assume the accreditation role. In the mid-1980s, the IOC recruited a number of laboratories to carry out drug testing worldwide. The initial IOC laboratory "accreditation" process began in 1985. In 1998, the Olympic Movement Anti-Doping Code (OMADC) was drafted, which established a more rigorous legal basis for the anti-doping process. The purpose of testing was not simply to catch cheaters, but rather to deter the use of performance-enhancing drugs.

In 1999, the World Anti-Doping Agency (WADA) was created to promote, coordinate and monitor the fight against doping. Unlike earlier anti-doping efforts, WADA is an independent agency. The sports movement, including the IOC, and governments fund WADA equally and are represented equally on the WADA Foundation Board. WADA coordinated the development and implementation of the World Anti-Doping Program, which was approved at an international congress in Helsinki in 2002. It consists of the World Anti-Doping Code (Code),[1] the List of Prohibited Substances and Methods (List),[2] the International Standard for Testing (IST),[3] the International Standard for Laboratories (ISL)[4] and the International Standard for Therapeutic Use Exemptions. The Code and several of the International Standards were modified and approved at a second international congress in Madrid in

2007. The new version of the Code will go into effect in January 2009. Since governmental bodies cannot sign treaties with nongovernmental entities, the governments have signed a United Nations Educational Scientific and Cultural Organization (UNESCO) international convention effective in February 2007 to adopt the essential elements of the Code into national laws.[5]

The Code sets out the anti-doping rules and principles, establishes the role of education and research in the anti-doping area, defines the roles and responsibilities of various stakeholders, and provides guidelines for implementation, modification, and compliance of signatories with the Code. With respect to the analysis of samples, the Code mandates that the analysis be performed in a WADA-approved laboratory. Further, the Code defines doping as detection by the laboratory of any amount of a prohibited substance or its metabolites or its markers in an athlete's sample. Only those substances naturally found in the body that have a reporting threshold established in the List are exceptions to this rule. Thus, for most doping violations, the laboratory must identify, but not quantify, the prohibited substance, metabolite or marker. The Code also provides that the athlete whose sample has an adverse analytical finding has a right to a hearing to address whether a doping violation occurred and the appropriate consequences. In the United States, the Ted Stevens Amateur Sports Act provides that matters related to an athlete's eligibility are to be heard by the American Arbitration Association (AAA). The protocols of the United States Anti-Doping Agency (USADA) establish that arbiters appointed to hear doping cases must be members of both the AAA and the Court of Arbitration for Sport (CAS). This is a good illustration of how national law interacts with the rules and procedures of sport and the need for the UNESCO convention.

Having established the right of an athlete to a hearing process, the Code also lays out the procedures to be used in establishing a doping offense.

> Anti-doping rules, like competition rules, are sport rules governing the conditions under which the sport is played. *Athletes accept these rules as a condition of participation* [emphasis added]. Anti-doping rules are not intended to be subject to or limited by the requirements and legal standards applicable to criminal proceedings or employment matters.
>
> (Reference (1), p. 7)

> 3.1 Burdens and Standards of Proof
>   The Anti-Doping Organization shall have the burden of establishing that an anti-doping rule violation has occurred. The standard of proof shall be whether the Anti-Doping Organization has established an anti-doping rule violation to the comfortable satisfaction of the hearing body bearing in mind the seriousness of the allegation which is made. This standard of proof in all cases is greater than a mere balance of probability but less than proof beyond a reasonable doubt.
>
> (Reference (1), p. 12)

This burden of proof is consistent with that applied to professional misconduct in many countries. It is not necessary within the anti-doping rules to establish intent, a concept called strict liability. This, along with other provisions of the Code (for example, the fact that there can be no challenge to the inclusion of a substance on the List), makes attack on the laboratory results the main defense strategy in any arbitration hearing. All of this is relevant to the laboratory in deciding whether a particular method used for detection of a prohibited substance is "fit for purpose."

The ISL establishes the rules and responsibilities of the laboratories in testing for substances contained on the List. As will be described in more detail, the ISL is an application of the ISO/IEC 1725 Standard to the field of antidoping testing. As such, it expands on the requirements of the laboratory to deal with issues such as receipt and retention of urine and blood samples, initial versus confirmatory tests, split sample (i.e. "A" and "B" bottle) testing, and other issues that are specific to anti-doping testing. The IST sets out rules to ensure that the collection of samples is uniform.

2 Analytical challenges in testing for performance-enhancing substances

The first analytical challenge is the composition of the List. The List prohibits the use of five classes of substances at all times: anabolic agents including endogenous and exogenous steroids and related substances; hormones and related substances such as growth hormone, erythropoietin, and insulin; β_2-agonists; agents with anti-estrogenic activity such as aromatase inhibitors and selective estrogen receptor modulators; and diuretics and other masking agents. Methods prohibited at all times are enhancement of oxygen transport by methods such as blood doping; chemical and physical manipulation of the sample; and gene doping. In addition, the List prohibits the use of stimulants, narcotics, cannabinoids and glucocorticosteroids when the athlete is tested at a competition. The List is an "open list," meaning that it incorporates not only the substances listed by name as examples, but also substances that are not listed by name but have similar chemical structures or pharmacological activities. Thus, for example, when an athlete's urine sample was found to contain the stimulant modafinil, not only was the laboratory expected to test for it, but a portion of the arbitration case involved proving that modafinil was related to other stimulants listed as examples by name on the List. In addition to an ever-increasing list of therapeutic agents that can be abused, the potential for "designer drugs," such as tetrahydrogestrinone (THG), requires that the laboratories be vigilant in their testing schemes. This requires that the "fitness for purpose" of a test for anti-doping be carefully considered. One can contrast the need for identifying new abuse substances, for example, with the situation in workplace testing for drugs of abuse, where the analyte menu and procedures are tightly defined and the testing has become essentially a commodity.

As has occurred in many fields of scientific endeavor, the development of reliable analytical tools has preceded advances in detection, measurement and interpretation in anti-doping. The first testing at an Olympic Games occurred in Mexico City in 1968. At the 1972 Munich Olympics, Manfred Donike used gas chromatography in combination with a nitrogen-selective detector for analysis of stimulants. Testing for anabolic steroids using radioimmunoassay, a technique invented in 1960, occurred at the Montreal Olympic Games in 1976. A major step forward occurred in 1983 with the commercial development of the capillary gas chromatograph interfaced with a bench-top quadrupole mass spectrometer (GC/MS). The application of this sensitive technique capable of identifying trace amounts of anabolic steroids resulted in a large number of last-minute withdrawals from competition and sanctions for anabolic steroid use at the Caracas Pan American Games. Improvements in the sensitivity of GC coupled to combustion/isotope ratio mass spectrometry (GC/C/IRMS) have made discrimination of pharmaceutical testosterone from natural testosterone on the basis of ^{13}C depletion possible.[6] Similarly, the development of high-performance liquid chromatography (HPLC) coupled to a tandem mass spectrometer (MS/MS) has made the detection of polar small molecules[7] and peptides and proteins[8,9] feasible. Thus, the analytical scope of testing in the anti-doping laboratories has broadened dramatically in the past decade.

The second analytical challenge arises from the fact that in anti-doping testing there is an active effort to avoid detection by some individuals who are being tested. For example, after the development of a urine test for recombinant erythropoietin (EPO), it was apparent from the isoelectric focusing patterns observed over time that some athletes changed from regular to micro-dosing in order to "beat the test." An advisory note, presumably from an athlete support person, further illustrates the active process of avoiding detection by advising:

> . . . so the first way to beat the test is to pee not a drop more than 75 ml [Note: 75 ml is the minimum volume of urine required in the IST] . . . with enough resources the exact dosage to be clear in 10 hrs or less could be determined quite easily. From this perspective it would seem the only rider ever caught using EPO, would be the ones unlucky enough not to have had the money to gain access to the top doctors and researchers working in labs to gain the knowledge of exact excretion rates.[10]

Because of the sample preparation technology used, a larger volume of urine could be used to compensate for a low concentration of EPO. Someone with sufficient expertise to realize that limiting the volume would mean that the laboratory could have an insufficient volume to confirm the initial test result provided the advice regarding the sample volume. Thus, the laboratories are constantly challenged to improve their limits of detection and identification or quantification, and to carefully manage the urine volume available to them. Athletes have also been known to attempt to manipulate or adulterate their urine samples with substances intended to mask their use of a prohibited substance. In the case of EPO, some athletes have attempted to add laundry detergent to their urine sample in the belief that the protease included in the detergent for stain removal would destroy any EPO in their sample.

Finally, the data produced by the anti-doping laboratories is to be used in an arbitration hearing to determine the athlete's eligibility to compete. The anti-doping rules, as established by the WADA Code, are incorporated into the rules of each individual sport. The athlete agrees to the anti-doping rules as a condition of competition in the same way that he or she agrees to play the game of basketball, for example, on a court of prescribed dimensions and with a basket of determined diameter whose rim is set at 10 feet.

3 The WADA laboratory system

Overseeing the performance of the laboratories in the anti-doping movement is a critical part of WADA's mission. The development of the WADA ISL was based on a number of important considerations. First, the international nature of sport and the global distribution of the recognized laboratories made the use of an internationally recognized accreditation process mandatory. Second, because of the rapidly changing landscape of doping, it was imperative to develop a system that could rapidly incorporate the newest advances in technology. Third, a balance needed to be achieved between the incorporation of new, potentially expensive and technically demanding methodologies, with the resulting differences in laboratory performance, and the equal treatment of athletes who could be tested in any of the WADA-recognized laboratories. Fourth, there was a need to put into place a proficiency testing system to assist the laboratories in achieving the performance goals established in the technical documents. Finally, the forensic nature of the scientific information produced by the laboratories needed to be recognized.

3.1 ISO/IEC 17025 and laboratory accreditation

Following the strategy of the IOC Sub-commission on Doping and Biochemistry in Sport implemented in 2000, WADA elected to have all of the recognized laboratories in the anti-doping system obtain ISO/IEC 17025 accreditation from the relevant national accrediting body as a prerequisite to obtaining or retaining WADA recognition. Accreditation, in contrast with certification, is often defined as "a formal recognition that an organization is competent to perform certain specified tasks."

> Laboratory accreditation bodies assess whether a laboratory meets certain criteria and the decision of an accreditation body to accredit a laboratory is thus *a statement of the competence of the laboratory* in a specific

technical area. But such a statement of competence does not mean that the accreditation body guarantees the validity of each and every test result.

(Reference[11], p. 18)

The ISO/IEC international standard[12] enumerates the management and technical requirements for the operation of a competent testing laboratory. Quality management aspects of the standard require policies, for example, for document handling, prevention and control of nonconforming work, and corrective actions. Technical requirements include personnel qualifications, appropriate laboratory space and equipment, selection and validation of test methods, measurement traceability, assuring the quality of test results, and reporting of test results. The ISO/IEC standard is written in general terms to cover testing that is not specifically chemically based, and thus implementation of the standard to chemical and biological testing laboratories requires a thorough understanding of the standard. ISO/IEC 17025 recognizes that each scientific discipline may have specific guidelines and requirements that are not enumerated in the general requirements for testing laboratories. The ISL was thus written as an *application* to the field of anti-doping as envisioned within Annex B of the ISO/IEC 17025 standard.

Keeping in mind the changing nature of doping strategies designed to beat the anti-doping testing system and the need to incorporate new technology, WADA has adopted the concept of performance-based methods as opposed to standardized methods. The limitations of standardized methods can be appreciated by reviewing the history of environmental testing industry, which is highly regulated by the US Environmental Protection Agency.[13] The basic concept of performance-based methods is for the regulatory body (e.g. WADA) to establish an acceptable level of method performance and allow the use of any method that meets that level of performance. This approach has laboratory accreditation implications since methods are developed in-house and thus require appropriate validation.

While WADA has retained the authority to site-visit any of the recognized laboratories,[4] the relevant national accrediting body handles the regular surveillance and assessment of the laboratory conformance with ISO/IEC 17025. WADA has worked with the International Laboratory Accreditation Cooperation (ILAC) to facilitate the concomitant assessment of the laboratories against the ISL by the relevant national accrediting body. In some parts of the world, the accrediting body that is the signatory to the ILAC convention may be in another country. The ILAC is a formal cooperation that establishes a network of mutual recognition agreements among accreditation bodies. The signatory national accrediting bodies have been peer-reviewed and shown to meet the ILAC's criteria for competence. Thus, laboratories around the world can be assessed and recognized as being competent within their scope of accreditation by means of a uniform system of assessment. This independent assessment of laboratory competence provides assurance for the athlete and other stakeholders of the quality of the global testing system.

3.2 *The ISL and technical documents*

The ISL[4] specifies defined terms, describes the WADA laboratory recognition process, and amplifies and clarifies the general laboratory requirements enumerated in ISO/IEC 17025. Despite its development primarily as an ISO/IEC 17025 application, the ISL has been used in three distinct ways:

1   as guidance for the laboratories in striving for uniform test performance and result reporting;
2   as a supplemental document against which the laboratory is assessed by their relevant national accrediting body; and
3   as a document that defines the requirements and responsibilities of the laboratory in performing testing on samples in the arbitration process.

Although applications to ISO/IEC 17025 are in general not stand-alone documents, WADA directed that the ISL be written as a stand-alone document following the model of the OMADC.[14]

In addition to the ISL, WADA has promulgated seven technical documents as guidance for the laboratories as a part of the system to achieve harmonized performance. The technical documents are required to be implemented by the laboratories as a part of the ISL. These documents provide guidance on laboratory chain of custody,[15] identification criteria for GC/MS and LC/MS methods,[16] documentation packages,[17] minimum required performance levels,[18] and reporting and evaluation guidance for endogenous steroids,[19] norandrosterone,[20] and recombinant erythropoietin (rEPO).[21]

3.2.1 *Setting performance goals*

WADA, through the Code, has the responsibility of establishing the performance goals on which the performance-based method rests. Specified characteristics of the methods could include limits of quantification and/or identification, linear dynamic range, specificity, and measurement uncertainty. Many of the current technical documents address performance goals. WADA TD2003IDCR[16] lays out the criteria for identification of compounds using GC/MS and HPLC/MS. The criteria in this document have been compared to those used in other fields[22] and found to be scientifically consistent. The next revision of this document will need to address method identification criteria for peptides and proteins.

The minimum required performance levels[18] set out the limits of identification for the classes of prohibited substances. Given the hundreds of substances (and their metabolites and markers) on the List, it should be recognized that a drug class-based approach has significant limitations. For example, both morphine and fentanyl are drugs within the narcotic class of prohibited substances, but the pharmacological potency and metabolic transformation of the two drugs result in urinary concentrations that differ by orders of magnitude. Thus, professional judgment of the accredited laboratory staff is necessary in establishing relevant reporting limits and methods that are fit for purpose.

Several of the technical documents set performance criteria for substances that are found naturally in the human body but also have the potential to be abused. The technical document on endogenous anabolic androgenic steroid testing and reporting provides a good example of the advances in results management in doping control and the evolution of performance criteria. Initially, the criterion for the detection of testosterone misuse was established through the measurement of the testosterone to epitestosterone (T/E) ratio in urine. The most frequently observed ratio was 1:1. Population studies demonstrated that T/E ratios greater than 6:1 occurred at a frequency of less than 1:5,000. Subsequently WADA decreased the threshold for T/E ratio to 4:1. But the use of population limits does not take into account that an individual with a natural T/E ratio of 0.1 could take a significant amount of testosterone before exceeding the threshold. In 1994, Donike and coworkers reported that intraindividual variability of the T/E ratio was much smaller than the population variance.[23] As a result, individuals with T/E ratios greater than the threshold had their values compared to either previous values or subsequent values (e.g. via longitudinal studies). If the values were not within 30 percent variation in men and 60 percent in women, the case was investigated further as a potential doping violation. The drawback to this approach was that the threshold had to be exceeded at least once to trigger the investigation. Recently, the laboratories have been asked to report steroid profile data to the responsible anti-doping agency. The agency uses computer databases and sophisticated methods of comparing longitudinal values from T/E ratio tests, such as the reference change value[24] and Bayesian[25] models, to determine individual thresholds for T/E ratio and other steroid concentrations. The individual reference range approach will significantly narrow the window available for doping. This will also require additional specification of laboratory performance and the fitness for purpose of the laboratory methods.

The urine "steroid profile" has been used to detect the administration of other anabolic steroids and precursors. For example, misuse of 5α-dihydrotestosterone would be manifested in 5α-metabolites (such as 5α-androstanediol), while the 5β-metabolites would not be affected. In addition, unique metabolites, such as the appearance of 6α-hydroxy-androstenedione after administration of androstenedione, appear in the urine after ingestion of large amounts of these natural substances. Similar approaches can be taken for dehydroepiandrosterone (DHEA) and other prohibited steroids found normally in the body.

Finally, the GC/C/IRMS technique has been used to detect testosterone and other "natural" substances originating from pharmaceutical products. The detection of a compound whose ^{13}C content is significantly different than that of an endogenous reference compound that reflects endogenous production is considered definitive evidence of doping. Unfortunately, a negative

GC/C/IRMS result is not definitive evidence for an athlete not having abused testosterone. The technical document addresses both required laboratory performance and results reporting issues.

3.2.2 Method development and validation

As was mentioned above, essentially all of the methods used in doping control are developed in individual laboratories. As a result, the analytical characteristics of the method must be verified during the research and development stages of its development. One of the initial steps in developing a method is establishing the performance characteristics, such as detection limit, linear dynamic range, precision and accuracy, necessary to have the analytical results support the intended use. This step is frequently referred to ensuring fitness for purpose. Validation of the method includes documenting that these analytical characteristics have been achieved. Guidance for some of the analytical characteristics is provided in the WADA technical documents.

Measurement uncertainty conveys the range of values that could reasonably be attributed to, for example, a concentration. It should be noted that uncertainty is associated with a particular measurement, not a method. Uncertainty among laboratories includes within-laboratory variance, between-laboratory variance, and bias. An estimate of the uncertainty should be initially obtained during method validation and should include components from different operators, equipment, reagents and calibration curves. Two approaches have been identified for estimation of quantitative measurement uncertainty: the bottom-up approach and the top-down approach. There have been relatively detailed discussions of the bottom-up, or uncertainty budget, approach, such as the Eurachem/CITAC Quantifying Uncertainty in Analytical Measurement document.[26] The top-down approach, favored by many in the analytical chemistry community,[27] involves the use of inter-laboratory studies to establish a system-wide value of uncertainty. Measurement uncertainty is a consideration in determining whether or not a result exceeds a reporting threshold.[28]

The scientific community has had a more difficult time achieving consensus on the issue of measurement uncertainty in qualitative analysis. Sphon[29] demonstrated that when three ions were detected within specified abundance criteria by mass spectrometry alone, diethylstilbestrol was the only compound that met those criteria in a database of 30,000 compounds. Stein and Heller[30] performed a similar study with a library of over 100,000 compounds and concluded that confidence improves with the inclusion of additional ions and that a full-scan spectrum is superior to selected ion monitoring if instrument sensitivity is adequate. Despite the fact that neither of these studies considered the selectivity added by sample preparation steps and the separating power of capillary gas chromatography or high-performance liquid chromatography, this empirical approach is the basis for most workplace, environmental, food and forensic testing at low concentrations. Recognizing that each step in the analytical method provides a degree of selectivity, Stephany and his colleagues in the animal residue analysis field proposed an "identification points" approach.[31,32] This has some appeal for the anti-doping field, particularly when one considers that the identification of several metabolites from the same prohibited substance would increase the certainty that it had been administered. The points approach might provide an easily understood way to combine these observations, especially when dealing with a legal environment with limited scientific expertise. A disadvantage of this approach is that for a particular matrix and a particular interference, a liquid–liquid extraction could be more effective than the small number of points allocated based on a global assessment of liquid–liquid extraction. For example, if hexane (as opposed to *tert*-butyl-methyl ether) is used as the organic phase in the method for norandrosterone, a metabolite of vitamin E that is not totally resolved by capillary gas chromatography is effectively removed. Thus, the actual impact on certainty is greater than that which would be assigned by global points system. It is thus difficult to create a simple system that reflects the analytical reality of the situation. Recently, a method for qualitative identification based on Bayesian statistics has also been proposed.[33,34] As scientific consensus is achieved regarding qualitative testing uncertainty, appropriate guidelines will be incorporated into the WADA ISL and technical documents.

3.3 Proficiency testing

The WADA Proficiency Testing program has been described.[35] The program has both educational and proficiency components. As new tests are added to the anti-doping armamentarium, educational round-robin tests assist in ensuring that the laboratories can obtain consistent results. The quarterly single-blind proficiency tests provide the laboratories with an opportunity to evaluate the results of their methodology against those of other anti-doping laboratories. In addition, documentation supporting the finding of a prohibited substance was reviewed and feedback provided to each laboratory. In 2006, WADA began a double-blind proficiency-testing program. In this program, proficiency-testing samples are submitted to the laboratory through routine collection channels, and the laboratory is not aware that the sample is part of a proficiency-testing program. In addition to WADA proficiency testing, the World Association of Anti-Doping Scientists (WAADS) has distributed educational round-robin tests to the WADA-recognized laboratories.

In summary, the WADA World Anti-Doping Program provides a framework for a unified global fight against doping. The WADA-recognized laboratories are a critical element in the program. Through the promulgation of laboratory standards and technical documents, a uniform system for laboratory testing has been established. The laboratories have annual surveillance for compliance with ISO/IEC 17025 and ISL international standards. Significant progress has been made over the past five years in harmonizing and improving laboratory performance.

The opinions expressed in this chapter are solely those of the author and do not represent the official positions, policies, or protocols of USADA, WADA, or any other agency with which the author may work.

4 References

1 WADA. *World Anti-Doping Code*, version 2.0. Available from http://www. wada-ama.org/rtecontent/document/code_v3.pdf (accessed November 16, 2007).
2 WADA. *The 2007 Prohibited List International Standard*. Available from http:// www.wada-ama.org/rtecontent/document/2007_List_En.pdf (accessed November 16, 2007).
3 WADA. *International Standard for Testing*, version 3.0. Available from http://www. wada-ama.org/rtecontent/document/testing_v3_a.pdf (accessed November 16, 2007).
4 WADA. *International Standard for Laboratories*, version 4.0. Available from http:// www.wada-ama.org/rtecontent/document/lab_aug_04.pdf (accessed November 16, 2007); WADA. *International Standard for Laboratories*, version 5.0. http:// www.wada-ama.org/rtecontent/document/lab_aug_04.pdf (accessed 16 December 2007).
5 United Nations Education Science and Cultural Organization. *International Convention Against Doping in Sport*. 2005. Available from http://portal.unesco.org/ en/ev.php-URL_ID=31037&URL_DO=DO_TOPIC&URL_SECTION=201.html (accessed November 16, 2007).
6 Shackleton CH, Phillips A, Chang T, Li Y. Confirming testosterone administration by isotope ratio mass spectrometric analysis of urinary androstanediols. *Steroids*. 1997; 62: 379–87.
7 Borts DJ, Bowers LD. Direct measurement of urinary testosterone and epitestosterone conjugates using high-performance liquid chromatography/tandem mass spectrometry. *Journal of Mass Spectrometry* 2000; 35: 50–61.
8 Liu C, Bowers LD. Mass spectrometric characterization of the beta-subunit of human chorionic gonadotropin. *Journal of Mass Spectrometry*. 1997; 32: 33–42.
9 Thevis M, Thomas A, Delahaut P, Bosseloir A, Schänzer W. Qualitative determination of synthetic analogues of insulin in human plasma by immunoaffinity purification and liquid chromatography-tandem mass spectrometry for doping control purposes. *Analytical Chemistry*. 2005; 77: 3579–85.
10 Anonymous document sent to USADA.
11 ILAC Document ILAC-I1:1994. *Legal Liability in Testing*. Available from http://www.ilac.org/home.html (accessed November 16, 2007).
12 ISO/IEC 17025:2005. *General requirements for the competence of testing and calibration laboratories*. International Organization for Standardization, Geneva, 2005.
13 Kimbrough DE, Spinner R. Performance based methods for regulatory analytical environmental chemistry: theory and practice. *American Environmental Laboratory*. 1994 November/December: 1–9.
14 *Olympic Movement Anti-Doping Code*. International Olympic Committee, Lausanne, Switzerland, 1999.
15 WADA Technical Document TD2003LCOC. Laboratory internal chain of custody. Available from http://www.wada-ama.org/rtecontent/document/chain_custody_1_2. pdf (accessed November 16, 2007).

16 WADA Technical Document TD2003IDCR. Identification criteria for qualitative assays incorporating chromatography and mass spectrometry. 2003. Available from http://www.wada-ama.org/rtecontent/document/criteria_1_2.pdf (accessed November 16, 2007).

17 WADA Technical Document TD2003LDOC. Laboratory documentation packages. 2003. Available from http://www.wada-ama.org/rtecontent/document/lab_docs_1_3.pdf (accessed November 16, 2007).

18 WADA Technical Document TD2004MRPL. Minimum required performance limits for detection of prohibited substances. 2004. Available from http://www.wada-ama.org/rtecontent/document/perf_limits_2.pdf (accessed November 16, 2007).

19 WADA Technical Document TD2004EAAS. Reporting and evaluation guidelines for testosterone, epitestosterone, T/E ratio, and other endogenous steroids. 2004. Available from http://www.wada-ama.org/rtecontent/document/end_steroids_aug_04.pdf (accessed November 16, 2007).

20 WADA Technical Document TD2004NA. Reporting norandrosterone findings. 2004. Available from http://www.wada-ama.org/rtecontent/document/nandrolone_aug_04.pdf (accessed November 16, 2007).

21 WADA Technical Document TD2007EPO. Harmonization of the method for the identification of epoetin alfa and beta (rEPO) and darbepoetin alfa (NESP) by IEF-double blotting and chemiluminescent detection. 2007. Available from http://www.wada-ama.org/rtecontent/document/td2007epo_en.pdf (accessed November 16, 2007).

22 Betham R, Boison J, Heller D, Lehotay S, Loo J, Musser S, Price P, Stein S. Establishing the fitness for purpose of mass spectrometric methods. *Journal of the American Society for Mass Spectrometry.* 2003; 14: 528–41.

23 Donike M, Rauth S, Mareck-Engelke U, Geyer H, Nitsche R. Evaluation of longitudinal studies, the determination of subject-based reference ranges of the testosterone/epitestosterone ratio. In: Donike M, Geyer H, Gotzmann A, Mareck-Engelke U, Rauth S, eds. *Recent advances in doping analysis: Proceedings of the Eleventh Cologne Workshop on Dope Analysis.* Cologne: Sport und Buch Strauß, 1994; 33–40.

24 Harris EK, Boyd JC. *Statistical bases of reference values in laboratory medicine.* New York: Marcel Dekker, 1995.

25 Sottas PE, Baume N, Saudan C, Schweizer C, Kamber M, Saugy M. Bayesian detection of abnormal values in longitudinal biomarkers with an application to T/E ratio. *Biostatistics.* 2007; 8: 285–96.

26 EURACHEM/CITAC Guide CG 4. *Quantifying uncertainty in analytical measurement.* 2nd ed. Available from http://www.eurachem.org/guides/QUAM2000-1.pdf (accessed November 16, 2007).

27 Analytical Methods Committee. Uncertainty of measurement: implications of its use in analytical science. *Analyst* 1995; 120: 2303–8.

28 EURACHEM/CITAC Guide. *Use of uncertainty information in compliance assessment.* 1st ed. 2007. Available from http://www.eurachem.org/ (accessed November 16, 2007).

29 Sphon JA. Use of mass spectrometry or confirmation of animal drug residues. *Journal of the Association of Official Analytical Chemists* 1978; 61: 1247–52.

30 Stein SE, Heller, DN. On the risk of false positive identification using multiple ion monitoring in qualitative mass spectrometry: large scale intercomparisons with a

comprehensive mass spectral library. *Journal of the American Society of Mass Spectrometry*. 2006; 17: 823–35.

31 André, F, De Wasch KKG, De Brabander HF, Impens SR, Stolker LAM, van Ginkel L, Stephany RW, Schilt R, Courtheyn D, Bonnaire Y, Fürst P, Gowik P, Kennedy G, Kuhn T, Moretain J.-P, Sauer M. Trends in the identification of organic residues and contaminants: EC regulations under revision. *Trends in Analytical Chemistry*. 2001; 20: 435–45.

32 European Community Decision 2002/657/EC of August 12, 2002 implementing Council Directive 96/23/EC concerning the performance of analytical methods and the interpretation of results. *Official Journal of the European Communities*. 2002; 221: 8–36.

33 Ellison SLR, Gregory S, Hardcastle WA. Quantifying uncertainty in qualitative analysis. *Analyst*. 1998; 123: 1155–61.

34 Mil'man BL. Identification of chemical compounds. *Trends in Analytical Chemistry*. 2005; 24: 493–508.

35 Ivanova V, Boghosian T, Rabin O. The WADA Proficiency Testing Program as an integral part of the fight against doping in sport. *Accreditation and Quality Assurance*. 2007; 12: 491–3.

3 Anabolic-androgenic steroids

Historical background, physiology, typical use and side effects

Richard V Clark

1 Introduction

This chapter will provide an overview of a very broad topic that spans decades of drug development on androgens, of research studies on the mechanism of action of anabolic-androgenic steroids (AAS), and of the purposeful, uncontrolled use by athletes seeking performance enhancement. There are several useful reviews of this topic that provide complementary information.[1-5] This review will discuss in more detail the physiological effects of AAS, especially relative to muscle effects, the medically appropriate and beneficial uses of testosterone and AAS, the abuse of AAS for gain in athletic performance, and the side effects of AAS.

2 Historical background: Discovery and development of anabolic steroids

The virilizing effects of the testis have been recognized by most societies for millennia, especially the critical role of the testis in puberty, the development of manhood and the effects of castration (causing eunuchoidism). Initial recorded proof of the virilizing effects of the testis was made in 1771 by John Hunter,[6] who induced male features in hens by the transplantation of testes from roosters. Later, Berthold[6] showed in 1869 that reimplantation of testes into castrate roosters prevented the loss of male characteristics. This study was the first published evidence that a single organ produced material that could affect the whole body; that is, an endocrine gland. Extrapolating from this discovery, the concept developed that the frailty linked with aging in men was related to failure of testicular function. This speculation led the renowned French physiologist Charles-Édouard Brown-Séquard to investigate the effects of extracts from dog and guinea pig testes. From studies based on self-administration, he reported beneficial effects on vigor, strength, intellect, and sexual potency.[7] While the aqueous extract probably had minimal activity, his stature in the scientific community gave credence to his allegations and stimulated great interest in the possibility of treating aging, and helped spur the discoveries of other hormones and endocrine glands.

Androgenic steroids were first isolated from urine using a biological assay, growth of a rooster's comb. The first androgenic steroid to be isolated was androsterone by Butenandt,[8] from 15,000 liters of male bovine urine. Previously, Loewe had shown that a testicular extract could stimulate growth of the seminal vesicle.[9] Testosterone was isolated from testicular extracts by Laqueur's group,[10] and, separately, synthesized by Ruzicka and Wettstein.[11] The anabolic effects of androgen extracts from urine were first demonstrated by Kochakian and Murlin, who showed that these caused nitrogen retention, an anabolic action rather than an androgenic effect.[12] Papanicolaou and Falk showed the dependence of skeletal muscle size in guinea pigs on androgens demonstrated by castration and replacement with testosterone proprionate.[13] And Kenyon's group showed a dose response for testosterone propionate for nitrogen retention and weight gain.[14]

These and similar studies at the time established that androgens show both androgenic and anabolic properties. "Androgenic" means masculinizing, inducing those body changes associated with testosterone which produce the male phenotype, including development of the secondary sex organs and growth of the penis, development of facial and body hair (especially axillary and pubic hair), vocal cord thickening and laryngeal enlargement leading to deeper voice, and the development of libido and sexual potency. "Anabolic" refers to the induction of growth and protein synthesis – that is, anabolism – such as muscle growth with increased muscle mass and strength, and bone growth with increased bone density and strength. Other compounds too, such as growth hormone, can have anabolic effects. Both androgenic and anabolic effects are dramatically demonstrated during puberty in young men, as they progress from boys to masculinized, muscular young men over a period of few years, induced by the endogenous androgens, primarily testosterone.

However, after the discovery of testosterone, plain crystalline testosterone was quickly recognized to have a short duration of exposure, only a few hours, regardless of whether it was administered orally, intramuscularly (IM), or intravenously. A variety of synthetic molecules were developed to provide a longer duration of action or to allow oral administration. The synthetic androgens were based primarily on substitutions on the D ring of native testosterone, either esterification at the 17-β-hydroxy group, or alkylation at the 17-α position. The esters are typically more potent than testosterone, with a much longer duration of action, being formulated as oil-based solutions.[15,16] They are given as IM depot injections, typically every one to four weeks (Table 3.1; testosterone cypionate, testosterone enanthate and nandrolone). The alkylated forms are less potent, but can be given orally (methyltestosterone, fluoxymesterone and oxandrolone). While initially popular, because they were delivered orally, the alkylated forms were found to cause serious liver injury, and their use is now discouraged.[2,3] The injectable ester forms were the dominant form of administration until the late 1990s, when topical preparations became available. Initially these were patches that were somewhat awkward to use and induced skin reactions. Later, in 2000, a gel was developed and introduced in the United States.[17,18] This has the advantage of avoiding IM injections, but must be applied once or twice daily, and can be transferred by personal contact. In the United States, the licensed market is split roughly 45 percent each between depot esters and gels. In Europe, an oral preparation of testosterone undecanoate (Andriol) is available, but must be taken at least twice a day with fatty food for adequate absorption, and has associated gastrointestinal side effects such as flatulence and loose stools. A long-acting depot formulation of testosterone undecanoate has recently become available in Europe, and is under review in the United States.[19] The major licensed forms of testosterone are shown in Table 3.1.

In addition to the licensed forms of testosterone, numerous alternative forms of AAS have been developed. The majority of these were created by ethical pharmaceutical companies and never advanced because of toxicological issues or poor pharmacokinetic characteristics, or because they simply did not offer advantages over the existing licensed products. However, many have been developed by illicit manufacturers specifically for unlicensed, unapproved distribution, that is the "black market," by copying or modifying known formulations These two sources differ greatly in their use. Licensed prescription of testosterone or AAS is typically done in a careful manner,

Table 3.1 Currently available anabolic androgenic steroids

	Brand name	Route of administration
Testosterone – unmodified		
Transdermal testosterone	Androgel, Testim	Dermal gel
	Striant	Buccal pellet
	Androderm, Testoderm	Dermal patch
Testosterone derivatives		
17-Hydroxyl esters		
Testosterone propionate		IM injection
Testosterone enanthate	Delatestryl	IM injection
Testosterone cypionate	Depo-Testosterone	IM injection
Testosterone undeconoate	Nebido	IM injection
Testosterone undeconoate[a]	Andriol	Oral
Nandrolone phenpropionate	Durabolin, Hybolin	IM injection
Nandrolone decanoate	Deca-Durabolin, Hybolin-D	IM injection
17-Alkylation		
Methyltestosterone	Android, Testred, Virilon	Oral
Fluoxymesterone	Halotestin	Oral
Oxandrolone	Oxandrin	Oral
Stanazol	Winstrol	Oral
Danazol	Danocrine	Oral
Other derivatives		
Mesterolone[a]	Mestoranum	Oral
Dihydrotesterone[a]	Andractim	Dermal gel

a Not available in the United States.

with appropriate doses. However, licensed compounds can be inappropriately prescribed, at excessive doses, leading to both a health problem and a source of abuse. The use of unlicensed compounds raises serious concerns at many levels, beginning with the lack of demonstration of safety of the compound in preclinical toxicology studies or in clinical trials as required for regulatory approval, and extending to the lack of quality controls in the manufacturing process, possibly producing products from poorly characterized compounds that may have variability in content and may contain potentially harmful contaminants.

Reports of inappropriate use of AAS to enhance athletic performance – doping – began as early as the late 1930s.[20] Definite AAS use in major international competition seems to have started at the World Weightlifting Championships in 1954, and then spread to other sports and the Olympics by the 1960s.[21,22] In the United States, this led to the Anabolic Steroid Control Act of 1990, which made it a felony to possess or distribute AAS for non-medical purposes. This Act also made AAS controlled substances, Class III, because of their abuse potential. However, the Dietary Supplement Health and Education Act of 1994 allowed preparations containing the androgens dehydroepiandrosterone (DHEA) and androstenedione to be considered "dietary supplements," though both of these are converted in the body to testosterone. Growth hormone (recombinant human growth hormone, rhGH) is a more recent entry to the anabolic agent class, increasing in use since the late 1990s, and will be discussed in Chapter 10.

3 Physiology: How AAS promote muscle growth

AAS have been clearly shown to stimulate muscle growth and increase muscle strength.[23-27] There are multiple mechanisms involved, including stimulation of protein synthesis, reduction of protein catabolism, recruitment of satellite cells, production of cytokines including IGF-1, and increase in androgen receptors, all leading to increased muscle size and strength.[28-30] Clinical studies have been limited in size and scope by medical considerations over causing harm to the subjects. Athletes taking AAS for performance enhancement use doses that can be five to 30 times the physiologic replacement dose, and are typically a mix of two to five different compounds.[31] Such doses and combinations cannot be considered reasonable for appropriately conducted clinical studies.

However, some carefully conducted clinical studies have been done which demonstrate the effects of progressive dose increments on muscle size and strength. Forbes showed a positive dose-response relation for AAS.[23] Bhasin and his colleagues did a series of studies in men given supra-physiologic replacement with testosterone for ten weeks. The subjects showed significant increases in both muscle size and strength, similar to those brought about by resistant training alone, and the increases were accentuated when testosterone and training were combined.[24] This study was followed by studies in young and older men with induced hypogonadism, which demonstrated a positive linear dose response for muscle size and strength with testosterone in both populations escalating from subtherapeutic replacement to increments four- to sixfold over therapeutic doses.[25,27]

These studies all used standardized measures of muscle strength, and there are few studies that have tried to evaluate the effects of AAS on athletic per- formance, which is a much more integrated activity involving multiple muscle groups and neuronal input, with the specific key activities varying greatly between sports. An early review of 25 studies on the effects of AAS in athletes concluded that AAS alone was not significantly effective, but was beneficial when combined with exercise and protein nutrition.[32] A later meta-analysis of 16 acceptable studies showed that androgen administration to trained athletes induced about a 5 percent increase in strength.[33]

These assessments are further complicated by the possibility of differential responses among different muscle groups. Studies suggest that upper-limb and neck musculature respond more strongly to AAS than lower-limb muscle groups.[34,35] Different tissues show differential responses to androgens, though the androgen receptor appears to be common across cell and tissue types.[36,37] However, the transcriptional co-activators and co-repressors can differ, and these determine the response in different tissues, and may affect response in tissue subgroups as different muscle groups.[38,39]

4 Use of anabolic-androgenic steroids

The medical use of AAS has been the primary driver for the development of the array of compounds available. The major indications include treatment of male hypogonadism (i.e. overt testosterone deficiency); anemia associated with bone marrow failure, such as aplastic anemia; improved nitrogen reten- tion and protein synthesis in catabolic states, such as in the case of severe infections; post-surgery; HIV wasting; cancer cachexia; and the treatment of angioneurotic edema.[2,40–42]

4.1 Typical use in sport

Although the use of steroids for the enhancement of athletic performance has been either illegal or prohibited by various sports leagues and governing bodies for some time, much is known about how athletes use these drugs.[43] For example, there are numerous "how-to" manuals and websites detailing their use, and linking to illicit supply sources. In addition, the National Institute on Drug Abuse (NIDA) has issued a research report on anabolic steroid abuse.[44] These readily available materials provide valuable insight into the nature of steroid use by athletes.

Steroid use by athletes usually involves techniques known as "cycling" and "stacking." "Cycling" refers to the timing of steroid use. The perceived benefit is that after prolonged steroid use, the muscles' receptor sites fail to recognize the steroid, and fusing of satellite cells with muscle cell diminishes. If this occurs, the steroid may lose its effectiveness, and even large doses may not provide significant muscle gains. Accordingly, "on" and "off" cycles are designed to obtain maximum effect of steroid use by allowing the cells to become receptive to the effects of steroids once more. "Stacking" involves use of two or more drugs at the same time. It is based on the belief that the use of different compounds will saturate steroid receptors in the muscles and provide a synergistic effect. A recent internet study indicates that a typical steroid regimen involves three different agents with a typical cycle duration ranging from five to ten weeks. Cycling and stacking patterns are also thought to reduce the adverse side effects of illegal steroid use by minimizing both the duration of use and the dosage necessary to obtain maximum performance-enhancing results.[31]

The doses typically used by athletes are much higher than those that would be prescribed for any legitimate therapeutic use. Estimates of these supra-physiologic doses have been reported to be between five and 100 times greater than the level of testosterone naturally produced by the body. These higher doses have a progressive relationship to increases in lean body mass and also reflect the general notion that if a low dose is effective, then more must be better.

5 Adverse effects of anabolic steroids

5.1 Endocrine – reproductive function

The addition of an excess amount of anabolic androgenic steroids to the body has marked consequences for both men and women.[1-3] In both genders, there is a suppression of the normal function of the gonads (testis and ovary) by inhibition of the pulsatile signals from the hypothalamus and pituitary gland that simulate production of sex steroids and sperm or eggs by the testis or ovary. In men, the suppression of the testis can result in a reduction in sperm count to minimal levels, causing infertility.[45,46] Depending on the dose and type of anabolic steroid, and the duration of use, overt testicular shrinkage can also occur. The time to recovery after such over-suppression of testicular function can be many months or longer. The virilizing effects of AAS manifest in the adult male as acne, which can be severe, resulting from excess stimulation of sebaceous glands on both the face and the body, and an increase in body hair and acceleration of male-pattern balding in those men with genetic predisposition. In addition, the excess androgens may overly stimulate the prostate gland, leading to prostate enlargement, with associated symptoms of impaired urination and a long-term concern over prostate cancer. Paradoxically, breast enlargement, gynecomastia, can occur as the body converts the excess testosterone or precursors to estradiol via the aromatase enzyme pathway, sometimes stimulating residual latent breast tissue in men.[1,3] The consequent breast enlargement varies in severity, but can be striking. Some AAS abusers take additional medications to block the effect of estrogen, such as tamoxifen, an anti-estrogen.

In women, AAS can suppress ovarian function via the same hypothalamic-pituitary axis as that which regulates ovarian function.[47] This leads to impaired ovulation and irregular or absent menstrual cycles, with markedly reduced production of endogenous estrogen and impaired fertility. The recovery period for normal ovarian function is variable, and can be several months. In women, the imbalance of AAS tilts toward androgen excess, and breast shrinkage and virilization can occur. Virilization is common, and more dramatic in women, with not only acne but inappropriate facial and body hair, and male-pattern balding. Beyond effects on the skin, androgens cause male-like enlargement of the voice box (larynx), causing a deepening of the voice, and enlargement of the clitoris. Several of these virilizing effects can be permanent, especially the voice deepening, clitoral enlargement, and balding.

5.2 Liver damage

The use of oral anabolic steroids has been clearly associated with liver injury, causing impaired liver function, especially for filtration and secretion of metabolic waste products including bilirubin, with development of cholestasis and jaundice (impaired secretion of bile), and hepatocellular necrosis. Rarer events include peliosis hepaticus (hemorrhagic blood-filled cysts that can rupture), and hepatocellular tumors and cancer.[48–50] These events have been clearly associated with the oral, alkylated AAS, and this is highlighted by the occurrence in young men, otherwise healthy, who are abusing anabolic steroids.[51,52] The occurrence of these serious side effects appears related to dose and duration, except for peliosis hepaticus, which is rare and seems to occur sporadically. While there is evidence that abnormal liver function resulting from steroid use is reversible after discontinuation for a period of three months, recurrent use of high doses typical in cycling routines may carry a risk of serious liver disorders over the long term. The risk of liver injury with depot injections and the recent gel formulations of anabolic steroids appears to be minimal.

5.3 Cardiovascular disease

Steroid use is associated with increased risk of several types of cardiovascular disease and dysfunction.[53,54] The occurrence of these side effects is based primarily on published case reports in which the occurrence of myocardial infarctions in young to middle-aged bodybuilders or weight lifters is attributed to steroid use.[55,56] These case studies are not definitive and do not take into consideration the effects of diet, genetic predisposition for cardiovascular disease, the nature or extent of steroid use by these athletes, or the use of concurrent medications, especially adrenergic mimetics. Moreover, the case studies do not provide a single, identifiable link between steroid use and cardiovascular disease.

However, recent studies with tissue Doppler imaging of the heart do suggest a link between a type of enlargement of the heart associated with strength training coupled with steroid abuse resulting in impaired cardiac function.[57,58] This is different than the changes in the heart observed in endurance athletes not using steroids, who show a beneficial form of heart enlargement more commonly known as an "athletic heart." Another form of heart enlargement that is clearly ominous is hypertrophic cardiomyopathy, which is genetically based and has been estimated to affect 1 in 500 individuals.[59] This condition is particularly important in sports medicine because of the association of exercise-induced arrhythmias, which can lead to loss of consciousness or death. There is growing evidence that steroid abuse can increase the risk associated with this type of cardiomyopathy in athletes.

In addition, there are significant data linking steroid use with adverse changes in cholesterol levels. Various studies show a link between excessive doses of steroids and detrimental effects on cholesterol levels.[60,61] Most notably, these studies show a direct and significant link between levels of steroid use and reductions of high-density lipoprotein (HDL) and elevated levels of low-density lipoprotein (LDL). The reduction in HDL levels can be 40 percent to 70 percent, depending on the dose and type of anabolic steroid, with the most pronounced adverse effect coming from the use of oral anabolic steroids.[4,62] The steroid-induced changes in cholesterol levels may not, per se, lead to heart disease, since the increased risk seems to be temporary, as cholesterol levels generally return to normal or baseline levels once steroid use is discontinued.

These studies provide clear support for the conclusion that athletes using steroids are at increased risk of heart disease.[63] This increased risk may be accentuated for an athlete who has other cardiovascular abnormalities.

5.4 Psychiatric and behavioral effects

A common perception is that androgens cause behavorial changes, especially aggressiveness and hostility. Clinical studies using moderately supra-physiologic replacement have generally shown mild to moderate effects,[64] and a study by Pope et al.[65] showed significant increases in aggressiveness and mania scores, especially among some subjects, though no changes were observed in healthy men given supra-physiologic doses.[25] When athletes taking significantly higher doses are evaluated, more behavioral pathology is observed. In studies on bodybuilders and athletes taking excess AAS, Pope and Katz[66,67] observed a significant frequency of irritability, hypomania and mania, and depression ranging from 10 percent to 40 percent. Depression during withdrawal from high-dose regimens appears common, and rates of depression among AAS abusers were higher during withdrawal from steroids than when actively taking steroids, and included suicide attempts.[68] Although rates of actual suicides are difficult to estimate, one series of 43 forensically evaluated deaths among male steroid users found that 11 steroid users committed suicide, 9 were homicide victims, 12 suffered accidental deaths and 2 were indeterminate.[69]

In summary, there is strong evidence that excessive dosing with AAS causes behavioral changes ranging from hostile, aggressive behavior to mania and depression, and even psychotic episodes. Further, there appears to be a risk of dependence on AAS, as well as the use of other illicit drugs.[66,70,71]

6 Conclusions

The use of AAS for performance enhancement is a problem at all levels of sports, from elite athletes in international competition to rising young aspirants in youth programs or high school. The competitive edge these compounds can provide does not come without a cost. There are definite health risks that can affect users. Some of these are predictable and common, such as suppression of testicular or ovarian function, causing impairment of endogenous sex hormones and infertility. Other risks are more serious and may even be fatal, though these are uncommon or rare, such as hepatic and cardiac toxicity. The suggestion that the risks associated with these compounds are exaggerated belies our limited clinical data and may encourage inappropriate use. The combined programs of educational publicity plus diligent screening for doping highlight the serious concern raised by this problem and the efforts to discourage the use of androgenic anabolic steroids.

7 References

1 Wilson JD. Androgen abuse by athletes. *Endocrine Reviews*. 1988; 9: 181–99.
2 Bagatelle CJ, Bremner WJ. Androgens in men: uses and abuses. *New England Journal of Medicine*. 1996; 334: 707–14.
3 Matsumoto AM. Clinical use and abuse of androgens and antiandrogens. In: Becker KL, ed. *Principles and practice of endocrinology and metabolism*. 3rd ed. Philadelphia: Lippincott Williams & Wilkins, 2001; 1181–200.
4 Hartgens F, Kuipers H. Effects of androgenic-anabolic steroids in athletes. *Sports Medicine*. 2004; 34: 512–54.
5 Hoffman JR, Ratamess NA. Medical issues associated with anabolic steroid use: are they exaggerated? *Journal of Sports Science and Medicine*. 2006; 5: 182–93.
6 Forbes TR. Crowing hen: early observations on spontaneous sex reversal in birds. *Yale Journal of Biology and Medicine*. 1947; 19: 955–70.
7 Brown-Séquard C-E. Des effets produits chez l'homme par des injections souscutanées d'un liquide retiré des testicules frais de cobaye et de chien. *Comptes rendus hebdomadaires des séances de la Société de Biologie (Paris)*. 1889; 1: 420–30.
8 Butenandt A. Über die chemische Untersuchung der Sexualhormons. *Zeitschrift für angewandte Chemine*. 1931; 44: 905–908.
9 Loewe S, Voss HE. Der Stand der Erfassung des männlichen Sexualhormons. *Klinische Wochenschrift*. 1930; 9: 481–7.
10 David K, Dingemanse E, Freud J, Laqueur E. Über krystallinisches männliches Hormon aus Hoden (Testosteron), wirksamer als aus Harn oder aus Cholesterin

bereitetes Androsteron. *Hoppe-Seylers Zeitschrift für physiologische Chemine.* 1935; 233: 281.

11 Ruzicka L, Wettstein A. Synthetische Darstellung des Testishormons, Testosteron. *Helvatica Chimica Acta.* 1935; 18: 1264–75.

12 Kochakian CD, Murlin JR. The effect of male hormone on the protein and energy metabolism of castrate dogs. *Journal of Nutrition.* 1935; 10: 437.

13 Papanicolaou GN, Falk EA. General muscular hypertrophy induced by androgenic hormones. *Science.* 1938; 87: 238.

14 Knowlton K, Kenyon AT, Sandiford I, Loturin G, Fricker R. Comparative study of metabolic effects of estradiol benzoate and testosterone propionate in man. *Journal of Clinical Endocrinology and Metabolism.* 1942; 2: 671–84.

15 Snyder PJ, Lawrence DA. Treatment of male hypogonadism with testosterone enanthate. *Journal of Clinical Endocrinology and Metabolism.* 1980; 51: 1335–9.

16 Sokol RZ, Palacios A, Campfield LA, Saul C, Swerdloff RS. Comparison of the kinetics of injectable testosterone in eugonadal and hypogonadal men. *Fertility and Sterility.* 1982; 37: 425–30.

17 Wang C, Berman N, Longstreth JA, Chuapoco B, Hull L, Steiner B, Faulkner S, Dudley RE, Swerdloff RS. Pharmacokinetics of transdermal testosterone gel in hypogonadal men: application of gel at one site versus four sites. *Journal of Clinical Endocrinology and Metabolism.* 2000; 85: 964–9.

18 Wang C, Swerdloff RS, Iranmanesh A, Dobs A, Snyder PJ, Cunningham G, Matsumoto AM, Weber T, Berman N; Testosterone Gel Study Group. Transdermal testosterone gel improves sexual function, mood, muscle strength, and body composition parameters in hypogonadal men. *Journal of Clinical Endocrinology and Metabolism.* 2000; 85: 2839–53.

19 Schubert M, Minnemann T, Hübler D, Rouskova D, Christoph A, Oettel M, Ernst M, Mellinger U, Krone W, Jockenhövel F. Intramuscular testosterone undecanoate: pharmacokinetic aspects of a novel testosterone formulation during long-term treatment of men with hypogonadism. *Journal of Clinical Endocrinology and Metabolism.* 2004; 89: 5429–34.

20 Boje O. *Bulletin of the Health Organization of the League of Nations.* 1939; 8: 439–69.

21 Todd T. Anabolic steroids: the gremlins of sport. *Journal of Sport History.* 1987; 14: 87–107.

22 Yesalis CE, Courson SP, Wright J. History of anabolic steroid use in sport and exercise. In: Yesalis CE ed. *Introduction to anabolic steroids in sport and exercise.* 2nd ed. Champaign, IL: Human Kinetics, 2000; 51–71.

23 Forbes GB. The effect of anabolic steroids on lean body mass: the dose response curve. *Metabolism.* 1995; 34: 571–3.

24 Bhasin S, Storer TW, Berman N, Callegari C, Clevenger B, Phillips J, Bunnell TJ, Tricker R, Shirazi A, Casaburi R. The effects of supraphysiologic doses of testosterone on muscle size and strength in normal men. *New England Journal of Medicine.* 1996; 335: 1–7.

25 Bhasin S, Woodhouse L, Casaburi R, Singh AB, Bhasin D, Berman N, Chen X, Yarasheski KE, Magliano L, Dzekow C, Dzekow J, Bross R, Phillips J, Sinha-Hikim I, Shen R, Storer TW. Testosterone dose-response relationships in healthy young men. *American Journal of Physiology.* 2001; 281: E1172–E1181.

26 Herbst KL, Bhasin S. Testosterone action on skeletal muscle. *Current Opinion on Clinical Nutrition and Metabolic Care.* 2004; 7: 271–7.

27 Bhasin S, Woodhouse L, Casaburi R, Singh AB, Mac RP, Lee M, Yarasheski KE, Sinha-Hikim I, Dzekov C, Dzekov J, Magliano L, Storer TW. Older men are as responsive as young men to the anabolic effects of graded doses of testosterone on the skeletal muscle. *Journal of Clinical Endocrinology and Metabolism*. 2005; 90: 678–88.

28 Ferrando AA, Sheffield-Moore M, Yeckel CW, Gilkison C, Jiang J, Achacosa A, Lieberman SA, Tipton K, Wolfe RR, Urban RJ. Testosterone administration to older men improves muscle function: molecular and physiological mechanisms. *American Journal of Physiolgy*. 2002; 282: E601–E607.

29 Bhasin S, Taylor WE, Singh R, Artaza J, Sinha-Hikim I, Jasuja R, Choi H, Gonzalez-Cadavid NF. The mechanisms of androgen effects on body composition: mesenchymal pluripotent cell as the target of androgen action. *Journal of Gerontological Biological Science and Medical Science*. 2003; 58: M1103–M1110.

30 Chen Y, Zajac JD, MacLean HE. Androgen regulation of satellite cell function. *Journal of Endocrinology*. 2005; 186: 21–31.

31 Perry PJ, Lund BC, Deninger MJ, Kutscher EC, Schneider J. Anabolic steroid use in weightlifters and bodybuilders: an internet survey of drug utilization. *Clinical Journal of Sport Medicine*. 2005; 15: 326–30.

32 Haupt HA, Rovere GD. Anabolic steroids: a review of the literature. *American Journal of Sports Medicine*. 1984; 34: 69–84.

33 Elashoff JD, Jacknow AD, Shain SG, Braunstein GD. Effects of anabolic-androgenic steroids on muscular strength. *Annals of Internal Medicine*. 1991; 115: 387–93.

34 Giorgi A, Weatherby RP, Murphy PW. Muscular strength, body composition, and health responses to the use of testosterone enanthate: a double blind study. *Journal of Science and Medicine in Sport*. 1999; 2: 341–55.

35 Hartgens F, Van Marken Lichtenbelt WD, Ebbing S, Vollard N, Rietjens G, Kupers H. Body composition, anthropometry in bodybuilders: regional changes due to nandrolone decanoate administration. *International Journal of Sports Medicine*. 2001; 22: 235–41.

36 Zhou ZX, Wong CI, Sar M, Wilson EM. The androgen receptor: an overview. Recent *Progress in Hormone Research*. 1994; 49: 249–74.

37 Scheller A, Hughes E, Golden KL, Robins DM. Multiple receptor domains interact to permit or restrict androgen-specific gene interaction. *Journal of Biological Chemistry*. 1998; 273: 24216–22.

38 Heinlein CA, Chang C. Androgen receptor coregulators: an overview. *Endocrine Reviews*. 2002; 23: 175–200.

39 McEwan IJ. Molecular mechanisms of androgen receptor-mediated gene regulation: structure-function analysis of the AF-1 domain. *Endocrine-Related Cancer*. 2004; 11: 281–93.

40 Dobs AS. Is there a role for androgenic anabolic steroids in medical practice? *Journal of the American Medical Association*. 1999; 281: 1326–7.

41 Basaria S, Wahlstrom JT, Dobs AS. Anabolic-androgenic steroid therapy in the treatment of chronic diseases. *Journal of Clinical Endocrinology and Metabolism*. 2001; 86: 5108–17.

42 Orr R, Singh MF. The anabolic androgenic steroid oxandrolone in the treatment of wasting and catabolic disorder. *Drugs*. 2004; 64: 725–50.

43 Yesalis CE, Kennedy NJ, Kopstein AN, Bahrke MS. Anabolic-androgenic steroid

use in the United States. *Journal of the American Medical Association*. 1993; 270: 1217–21.

44 National Institute on Drug Abuse. Anabolic steroids: a threat to mind and body. NIH Publication No. 96–3721, 1996.

45 Anderson RA, Wu F., Comparison between testosterone enanthate induced azoospermia and oligospermia in a male contraceptive study II. *Journal of Clinical Endocrinology and Metabolism*. 1996; 81: 896–901.

46 Torres-Calleja J, González-Unzaga M, DeCelis-Carrillo R, Calzada-Sánchez L, Pedrón N. Effect of androgenic anabolic steroids on sperm quality and serum hormones in adult male body builders. *Life Science*. 2001; 68: 1769–74.

47 Chang RJ. Polycystic ovary syndrome and hyperandrogenic states. In: Strauss JF, Barbieri RL, eds. *Yen and Jaffe's Reproductive Endocrinology*. 5th ed. Philadelphia: Elsevier Saunders, 2004; 597–632.

48 Ishak KG, Zimmerman HJ. Hepatotoxic effects of the anabolic/androgenic steroids. *Seminars in Liver Disease*. 1987; 7: 230–6.

49 Soe KL, Gluud C. Liver pathology associated with the use of anabolic-androgenic steroids. *Liver*. 1992; 12: 73–9.

50 Socas L, Zumbado M, Pérez-Luzardo O, Ramos A, Pérez C, Hernández JR, Boada LD. Hepatocellular adenomas associated with anabolic androgenic steroid abuse in bodybuilders: a report on two cases and a review of the literature. *British Journal of Sports Medicine*. 2005; 39: e27.

51 Creagh TM, Rubin A, Evans DJ. Hepatic tumours induced by anabolic steroids in an athlete. *Journal of Clinical Pathology*. 1988; 41: 441–3.

52 Kosaka A, Hayakawa H, Kusagawa M, Takahashi H, Okamura K, Mizumoto R, Katsuta K. Hepatocellular carcinoma associated with anabolic steroid therapy. *Journal of Gastroenterology*. 1996; 31: 450–4.

53 Nieminen MS, Rämö MP, Viitasalo M, Heikkilä P, Karjalainen J, Mäntysaari M, Heikkilä J. Serious cardiovascular side effects of large doses of anabolic steroids in weight lifters. *European Heart Journal*. 1996; 17: 1576–83.

54 Fineschi V, Baroldi G, Monciotti F, Paglicci Reattelli L, Turillazzi E. Anabolic steroid abuse and cardiac sudden death: a pathologic study. *Archives of Pathology and Laboratory Medicine*. 2001; 125: 253–5.

55 Dickerman RD, Stevens QE, Schneider SJ. Sudden cardiac death in a 20-year old bodybuilder using anabolic steroids. *Cardiology*. 1995; 86: 172–3.

56 Hausmann R, Hammer S, Betz P. Performance enhancing drugs (doping agents) and sudden death: a case report and review of the literature. *International Journal of Legal Medicine*. 1998; 111: 261–4.

57 Nottin S, Nguyen LD, Terbah M, Obert P. Cardiovascular effects of androgenic anabolic steroids in male bodybuilders determined by tissue Doppler imaging. *American Journal of Cardiology*. 2006; 97: 912–15.

58 Krieg A, Scharhag J, Albers T, Kindermann W, Urhausen A. Cardiac tissue Doppler imaging in sports medicine. *Sports Medicine*. 2007; 37: 15–30.

59 Spirito P, Bellone P, Harris KM, Bernabo P, Bruzzi P, Maron BJ. Magnitude of left ventricular hypertrophy and risk of sudden death in hypertrophic cardiomy-opathy. *New England Journal of Medicine*. 2000; 342: 1778–85.

60 Lenders JWM, Demacker PNM, Jansen JS, Hoitsma VL, van't Laar A, Thien T. Deleterious effects of anabolic steroids on serum lipoproteins, blood pressure, and liver function in amateur bodybuilders. *International Journal of Sports Medicine*. 1988; 9: 22.

61 Glazer G. Atherogenic effects of anabolic steroids on serum lipid levels. *Archives of Internal Medicine.* 1991; 151: 1925–33.

62 Hurley BF, Seals DR, Hagberg JM, Goldberg AC, Ostrove SM, Holloszy JO, Wiest WG, Goldberg AP. High-density-lipoprotein cholesterol in bodybuilders v. powerlifters: negative effects of androgen use. *Journal of the American Medical Association.* 1984; 252: 507.

63 Parssinen M, Seppala T. Steroid use and long-term health risks in former athletes. *Sports Medicine.* 2002; 32: 83–94.

64 Bahrke MS, Wright JE, Strauss RH, Catlin DH. Psychological moods and subjectively perceived behavioral and somatic changes accompanying anabolic-androgenic steroid use. *American Journal of Sports Medicine.* 1992; 20: 717–24.

65 Pope Jr HG, Kouri EM, Hudson JI. Effects of supraphysiological doses of testosterone on mood and aggression in normal men: a randomized controlled trial. *Archives of General Psychiatry.* 2000; 57: 133–40.

66 Pope, HG Jr, Katz DL. Affective and psychotic symptoms associated with anabolic steroid use. *American Journal of Psychiatry.* 1988; 145: 487.

67 Pope HJ, Katz DL. Psychiatric and medical effects of anabolic-androgenic steroid use. *Archives of General Psychiatry.* 1994; 51: 375–82.

68 Malone DA, Dimeff RJ, Lombardo JA. Psychiatric effects and psychoactive substance use in anabolic-androgenic steroid users. *Clinical Journal of Sport Medicine.* 1995; 5: 25.

69 Thiblin I, Lindquist O, Rajs J. Causes and manner of death among users of anabolic androgenic steroids. *Journal of Forensic Sciences.* 2000; 45; 16–23.

70 Brower KF, Eliopulos GA, Blow FC, Catlin DH, Beresford TP. Evidence for physical and psychological dependence on anabolic-androgenic steroids in eight weightlifters. *American Journal of Psychiatry.* 1990; 147: 510–12.

71 Midgley SJ, Heather N, Davies JB. Dependence-producing potential of anabolic-androgenic steroids. *Addiction Research and Theory.* 1999; 7: 539–50.

4 Testing for anabolic agents

Christiane Ayotte

1 Introduction

The decision was taken, more than 40 years ago, to exclude doping from amateur sport. In order to do so, the International Olympic Committee formed a Medical Commission responsible for defining the substances prohibited during competition and for establishing a network of laboratories capable of testing athletes' specimens. At the time, given the existing technology and knowledge, only stimulants (mainly amphetamines) could be tested for. The development of immunoassays for 17α-methylated steroids and 19-norsteroids gave the first tool for detecting anabolic-androgenic steroids (AAS),[1,2] but the real breakthrough came from the commercialisation of highly efficient software-operated analytical instruments combining high-resolution gas chromatography and mass spectrometry, allowing the automated analysis of batches of samples with high sensitivity.

Elucidation of the metabolic pathways of all AAS occurred in the 1980s, and was aimed ultimately at identifying the more efficient markers of utilisation. Those would be not only the main urinary metabolite but also the most persistent one, which would make it possible to trace back an earlier administration.[3–8] For many years, the tests were based upon the research by GC/MS (at low and high resolution), commonly under electron impact ionisation, of target markers or metabolites at a level of detection of 1 ng/mL and less. Notwithstanding the sensitivity and specificity of GC/MS analyses at such levels, because steroids are excreted as conjugates in a very complex matrix, a rather extensive sample preparation is required. Typically, after a solid-phase extraction and enzymatic hydrolysis, the volatility and stability of steroid analytes are increased by converting the ketones and hydroxyl groups into trimethylsilyl (TMS) enols, ethers (persilylation). The mass spectra of TMS derivatives are informative: molecular ions or fragments corresponding to the loss of a methyl group are often present, along with other characteristic ones.

More recently, the direct identification of conjugated metabolites by the combination of liquid chromatography and tandem mass spectrometry (LC/MS/MS) has been reported more frequently with electrospray ionisation (ESI), and comprehensive screening and confirmation methods were designed around those techniques.[9–11]

The confirmation of the presence of a purely synthetic AAS is based upon the unequivocal identification of the substance itself or one of its metabolites in the athlete's sample. The full mass spectrum could be utilised to achieve identification, or, when the levels are close to the limit of detection, the results of the acquisition of selected characteristic ions (selective ion monitoring (SIM) mode). Negative controls and reference materials are employed in each confirmatory assay (positive controls); these can be authentic standards of the metabolites or a well-characterised collection of specimens from an administration study.

2 Structures and metabolites

The AAS, whether for human or veterinary usage, are functionalised androstane (C_{19}) or estrane (C_{18}) structures. Testosterone and nortestosterone possess a ketone at C-3 conjugated to a double bond at C-4 and a hydroxyl at C-17β (Figure 4.1). Alternatively, methyl groups are introduced in the C-1, C-2 or C-7 positions, the A-ring can be saturated, the double bond moved to C-1 (e.g. methenolone, mesterolone, drostanolone, mibolerone), or added to the conjugated ketone (e.g. boldenone), while highly conjugated structures also exist (e.g. trenbolone). The AAS are often alkylated at C-17α, most frequently by a methyl group (e.g. methyltestosterone, methandienone). Other modifications include the introduction of chlorine at C-4 (chlortestosterone), fluorine at C-9 and hydroxyl at C-11 (fluoxymesterone), the attachment of a pyrazole cycle to the A-ring (stanozolol) or its replacement by a lactone (oxandrolone), while trenbolone and tetrahydrogestrinone are highly conjugated structures.

Using 19-nortestosterone as an example, phase I biotransformations involve enzymes causing oxidation, reduction or hydroxylation, while conjugation is a phase II process. The 3- and 17-hydroxysteroid dehydrogenases and the 5α-,5β-reductases convert 19-nortestosterone in its three main metabolites, 19-norandrosterone, 19-noretiocholanolone and 19-norepiandrosterone (Figure 4.2). While the first two are mostly glucuroconjugated (UDPGT: uridine diphosphate glucuronyltransferase), the third of these, possessing a 3β-OH, 5α-H configuration, is almost exclusively excreted as the sulphate (sulphatase). Norandrosterone is the marker for the utilisation of related norsteroids.[12]

Generally, 17-alkylated steroids are extensively metabolised. Several metabolites excreted in the free, glucuro- or sulphoconjugated forms were identified in urine samples collected following the administration of methandienone (17β-hydroxy-17α-methylandrosta-1, 4-dien-3-one). Hydroxylation at C-6β and C-16, sequential reduction of A-ring 3-keto-1,4-diene functionality are some of the processes observed.[7,13,14] Epimerisation at C-17 occurs most probably in the urine specimen by the intermediate formation of a tertiary carbocation from the original 17β-*O*-sulphate metabolites.[15–17] One metabolite, 18-nor-17β-hydroxymethyl-17α-methylandrost-1,4,13-trien-3-one (*G* in Figure 4.3) is persistent, allowing longer detection periods.[8]

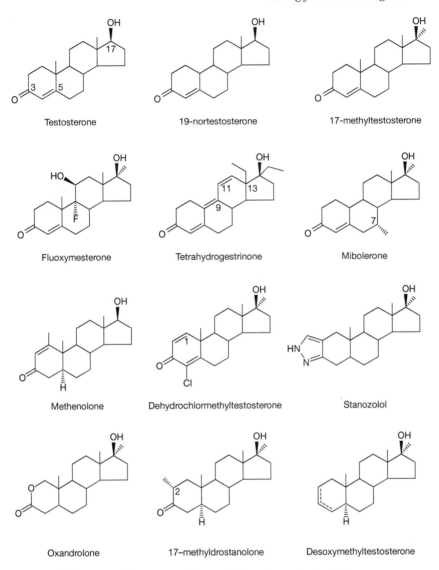

Figure 4.1 Structures of representative anabolic-androgenic steroids.

3 New steroids

Noticing the presence of new substances in athletes' samples is certainly a challenge to laboratories, and although several doping agents have been picked up throughout the years, many remained undetected. When a previously unknown product shows up in an athlete's sample, it must first be identified and its potential performance-enhancing or masking properties investigated. Some of the additions to the list of prohibited substances were in fact existing

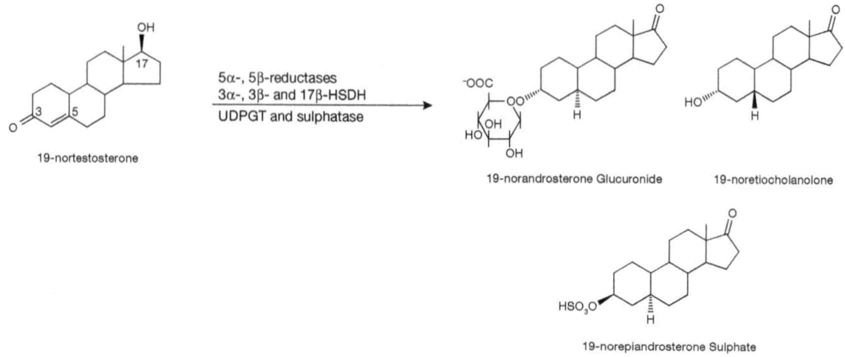

Figure 4.2 Biotransformation of 19-nortestosterone.

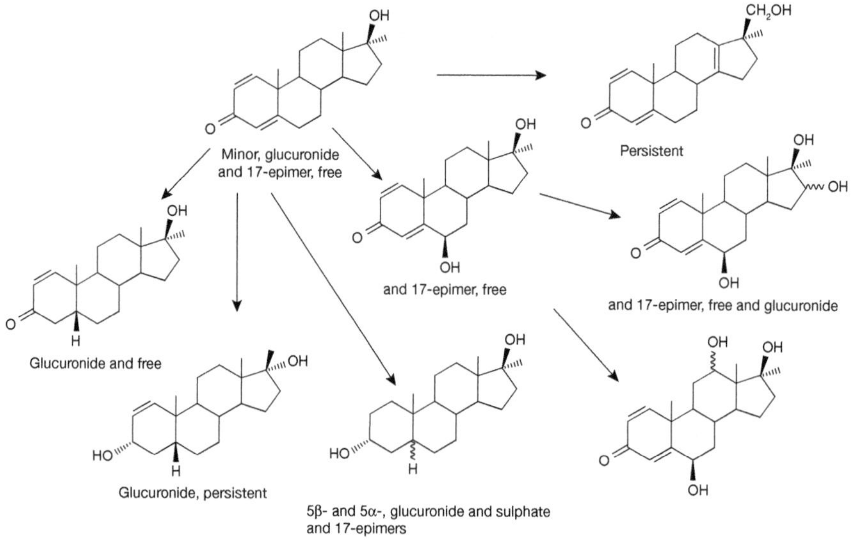

Figure 4.3 Biotransformation of methandienone.

Source: references 4–7.

human or veterinary medications that were believed to have performance-enhancing properties. Clenbuterol, a β_2-agonist, and zeranol, a veterinary non-steroidal growth promoter, were detected in samples in the early 1990s. A few years later, hard collective work was required to characterise the new molecules bromantan and carphedon, two stimulants produced by the Russian Pharmacology Institute and surreptitiously utilised by competing athletes who failed to mention them on their declaration form.[18]

During a period of almost ten years, as a direct consequence of the Dietary Supplement Health and Education Act adopted in the mid-1990s in the United States, new substances regularly and openly appeared on the market in products labelled with a rather confusing nomenclature and new terminology such as "pro-hormone" or "designer supplement." Others, more clandestinely shared, were characterised by anti-doping laboratories following seizures at customs, denunciations, or through the analysis of athletes' samples.

Steroids such as androstenedione (androst-4-en-3,17-dione) and dehydroepiandrosterone (DHEA) were referred to as testosterone pro-hormones, while others, such as boldione (androsta-1,4-dien-3,17-dione) and norandrostenedione (estr-4-en-3,17-dione or the delta-5 isomer), were related respectively to boldenone and to nandrolone (nortestosterone). Eventually it became possible to purchase "designer supplements", often new 17-alkylated steroids, for oral self-administration in spite of the total absence of quality controls and clinical studies that would have been required from the pharmaceutical industry. In that same period, a few athletes doped surreptitiously with the undetectable and secretly synthesised molecules norbolethone, tetrahydrogestrinone (THG) and desoxymethyltestosterone (DMT). While the first one was detected in an athlete's sample, the second one was handed out to sport authorities and the third one was seized at customs (Figure 4.4).

Counterfeit steroids must first be identified; once isolated from the raw preparation, structures are proposed from analyses by nuclear magnetic resonance and mass spectrometry. The full characterisation follows the synthesis of the authentic molecules and the correspondence of mass spectra and physicochemical properties.

With the aim of detecting with high sensitivity the markers of prohibited AAS, the GC or LC/MS first screening analysis looks for characteristic ions showing up at a defined retention time (SIM). In spite of this high specificity

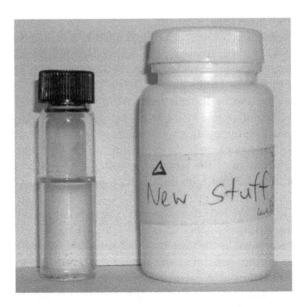

Figure 4.4 Clandestine steroid seized at the Canadian–US border. (The substance proved to be desoxymethyltestosterone.)

towards certain metabolites, it is nonetheless possible to pick up unknown steroids that would possess certain structural features such as a methyl group in the C-17 position, giving rise to an intense ion at m/z 143 in the mass spectrum of TMS derivatives, as long as the characteristic ions are monitored throughout the analysis. The same type of expanded screening assay has been proposed for ESI tandem mass spectrometry (combined to liquid chromatography).[11,19] Furthermore, the profile of endogenous steroid metabolites being carefully monitored during the screening assay, suppressed concentrations of final metabolites or altered ratios could be related to the administration of a synthetic AAS, which should lead to further investigations.

The characteristic and unusual ions at m/z 157 and 144 (17-ethylated D-ring fragmentation) of norbolethone (17β-hydroxy-18a-homo-19-nor-17α-pregn-4-en-3-one) and its putative metabolites were detected in two athletes' samples that raised suspicion owing to their significantly suppressed endogenous steroid profile.[20] The androgenic properties of norbolethone were investigated in the 1960s, but it was not marketed. Tetrahydrogestrinone (17β-hydroxy-18a-homo-19-nor-17α-pregna-4,9,11-trien-3-one), prepared from the chemical reduction of the 17-ethinyl group of gestrinone, a weak androgen with anti-estrogen and anti-progesterone activities, was identified in the raw preparation sent to the United States Anti-Doping Agency.[21] From different studies, THG, a purely counterfeit steroid, was shown to be a potent androgen anabolic agent,[22,23] and its detection in athletes' samples was hindered by its poor behaviour under the conditions of GC/MS analysis of TMS derivatives, multiple peaks being generated by the reagent employed. Tetrahydrogestrinone, a highly conjugated 3-keto-4,9,11-triene like trenbolone, is more compatible with liquid chromatography.

17α-Methyl-5α-androst-2-en-17β-ol and its 3-ene isomer (desoxymethyltestosterone, DMT) were rapidly synthesised and identified in a bottle of raw material labelled "New Stuff Δ" seized at the US–Canadian border in 2005. Identification was made by the material's characteristic ions at m/z 143 and 130 (17-methylated D-ring fragmentation) and single hydroxyl group.[24] The synthesis and the androgenic anabolic properties of DMT (Ergomax LMG, Phera-Plex) and 17α-methyldrostanolone, another designer steroid sold as Superdrol (methasterone), were described in the scientific literature of the 1960s.[25,26] The presence of the latter was spotted first in an athlete's sample along with other AAS. With characteristic ions at m/z 143 (17-methylated D-ring), 157, 141 (a methyl group at C-1 or C-2), the new steroid was found to be the 17α-methylated derivative of drostanolone (17β-hydroxy-2α-dimethyl-5α-androstan-3-one).[24]

The metabolites must be identified to allow detection. Since pharmaceutical-grade products are not accessible, the administration to human volunteers is restricted to the indispensable. *In vitro* studies with cryopreserved or fresh human hepatocytes afforded metabolic profiles that contain the metabolites excreted following the administration to volunteers of respectively, nortestosterone, drostanolone, methyldrostanolone[24] and androstenedione, norandrostenedione, tetrahydrogestrinone or gestrinone[27-29] as substrates. The potential of micro-somal and S9 fractions of human liver homogenates to produce the metabolites has also been investigated with 17-methylated models.[30] Optimally, the iden-tification of the metabolites thus generated is simplified by the absence of interferences inherent in the complex urine medium (Figure 4.5).

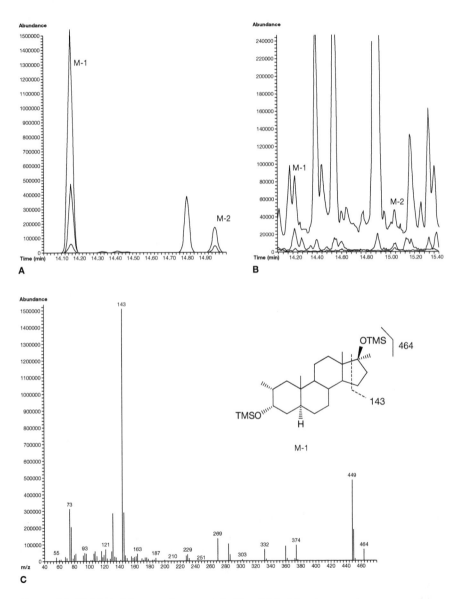

Figure 4.5 17-Methyldrostanolone metabolites M-1 (structure and mass spectrum (C)) and M-2 from the incubation of cryopreserved human hepatocytes (A) and human excretion study (B).

4 Detection of "natural" steroids

Detecting and confirming the administration of an anabolic androgenic steroid that could be present normally in the human body is complex and requires a careful evaluation of the profile of urinary metabolites. Testosterone (17β-hydroxyandrost-4-en-3-one) is available in a wide range of forms and dosages for oral, topical, transdermal administrations and intramuscular injections. The first probe for its detection, the increased ratio of urinary testosterone to epitestosterone (T/E value), was proposed in the early 1980s.[31] Both steroids are normally excreted as glucuronides and in equal proportion in males and females. The biological role of epitestosterone (17α-hydroxyandrost-4-en-3-one) is not fully known. It is not a metabolite of testosterone and its excretion can even be suppressed, although not systematically, following the repeated administration of some pharmaceutical preparations of testosterone.

The T/E values were measured in cohorts of thousands of male and female athletes' samples. While the majority are located at around 1, nearly one in 100 males and a few females normally and systematically produce samples with values of up to 10, which makes it impossible to rely solely on a single slightly high T/E value to prove the administration of testosterone.[32] Corroborative evidence is collected through the routine measurement of the concentrations and relative ratios of testosterone, epitestosterone, final and inactive metabolites, androsterone (5α-androstan-3α-ol-17-one), etiocholanolone (3α-hydroxy-5β-androstan-17-one), androstandiols (5α-androstan-3α,17β-diol and 5β-androstan-3α,17β-diol), which constitutes the individual steroid profile.

By the end of the 1990s, the results from carbon isotope ratio mass spectrometry (IRMS) were considered to provide direct evidence of the exogenous origin of urinary testosterone metabolites.[33-37] The GC/C/IRMS instrument combines gas chromatography (GC), combustion (C) and isotope ratio mass spectrometry (IRMS); typically, the steroids eluted from the gas chromatograph are converted to CO_2 by combustion, and the mass spectrometer is set to measure $^{13}C^{16}O_2$ (*m/z* 45) and $^{12}C^{16}O_2$ (*m/z* 44). The ratio is expressed as $\delta^{13}C$ (per mille) values. Steroids contained in pharmaceutical preparations or commercial products, such as androstenedione and DHEA, are not found in nature; they are prepared by chemical reactions on starting material, usually plant sterols. Since plants assimilate the carbon isotopes differently depending on their particular photosynthetic pathway (either C3, C4 or CAM), the $\delta^{13}C$ values of their sterols are typical. Most frequently, AAS originate from C3 plants, and as such they will show a clearly depleted ^{13}C content that is retained in all the metabolites produced and excreted following the administration of the synthetic AAS. Notwithstanding relatively minor individual differences that could be attributed to environmental factors and diet, the human steroids from normal metabolic processes are found at values differing significantly from those of "synthetic" steroids, with $\delta^{13}C$ values characteristic of food of mixed vegetal origin.

The GC/C/IRMS analyses are integral parts of the detection and confirmation of the administration of testosterone, of its active metabolite dihydrotestosterone (DHT, 17β-hydroxy-5α-androstan-3-one) and precursors, such as dehydroepiandrosterone (DHEA, 17β-hydroxyandrost-5-en-3-one), androstenedione (androst-4-ene-3,17-dione), as well as epitestosterone, which could be utilised as a masking agent (Figure 4.6).

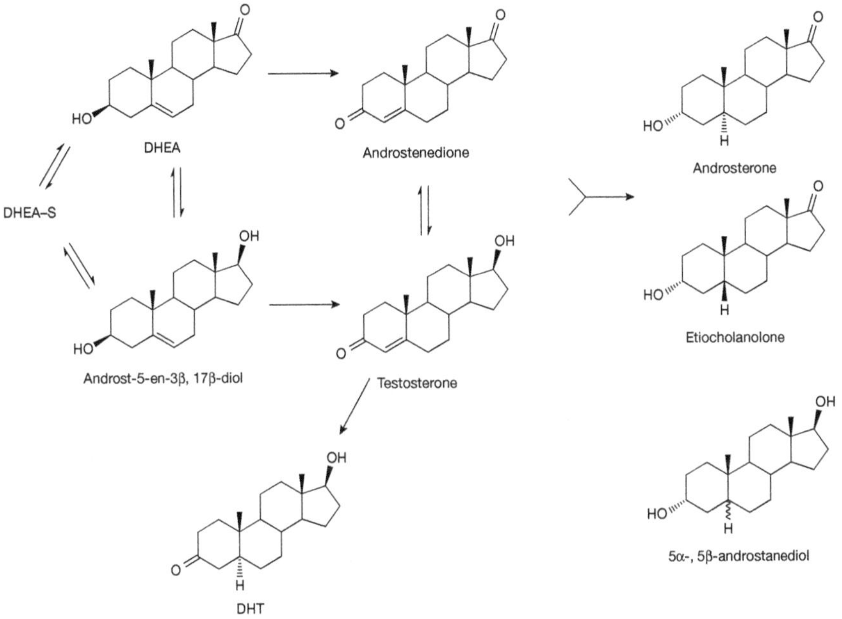

Figure 4.6 Relation between testosterone, its metabolites and precursors of interest.

5 Profiles of urinary steroids analysed by GC/MS and GC/C/IRMS

The selected metabolites, markers of the administration of potentially endogenous AAS, are measured by GC/MS analysis in the SIM mode of isolated extracts that were hydrolysed (β-glucuronidase) and converted to pertrimethylsilyl derivatives. Careful adjustment of the preparation and analytical conditions is crucial. The hydrolysis step must be free of side reactions and ensure the complete deconjugation of key steroids, while the quantitative assay must include appropriate internal standards, calibration curves and quality control samples. For example, only purified β-glucuronidase from *E. coli* should be employed, to maintain the integrity of the steroid profile. Undesirable side activities such as that of 3-hydroxysteroid dehydrogenase are present in other preparations such as crude mixtures of *Helix pomatia*, resulting in the conversion of androst-5-en-3,17-diol into testosterone. In cases when the analysis of the sulphoconjugated metabolites is required, only the sulphate of

DHEA is readily hydrolysed by the arylsulphatase contained in *H. pomatia* mixtures. Androsterone, testosterone and other sulphoconjugated metabolites require solvolysis for cleavage. With regard to the IRMS, the methods employed are generally based upon the analysis of fractions of metabolites purified by solid-phase extraction (SPE) or high-performance liquid chromatography (HPLC), injected as such or in the form of acetates. To compensate for individual variations and the different methodologies and instruments employed, the difference between each diagnostic metabolite, e.g. testosterone itself, androsterone, etiocholanolone, DHEA, 5α- and 5β-androstandiol and the other unaffected urinary steroids chosen as internal reference is determined (difference expressed as $\delta^{13}C$). Considering the normal variation, differences larger than three units for one or more metabolites are consistent with their being of exogenous origin.[38]

6 Variations of the T/E values and concentrations of urinary metabolites

Over the years, the statistical distributions of the several parameters of the urinary steroid profile have been determined in several thousand samples collected from male and female athletes of different origin and age, during training, rest and competition. Athletes' normal profiles are not unique; intense exercise and training do not appear to influence the excretion of testosterone and its principal metabolites. Starting with the T/E, first marker of the urinary steroid profiles, its distribution in major North American male and female athletes' samples analysed over a period of ten years confirms that, most frequently, the values are close to 1, with fewer than 1 percent being above 4.6 and 4.3 respectively. On that basis, a sample with a ratio greater than 4 is further analysed by GC/C/IRMS to determine whether the urinary metabolites are of exogenous or endogenous origin.[38] When all the other parameters of the steroid profile are within the ranges of values normally measured in humans, the case is concluded without having to conduct further follow-up testing.

The concentrations of excreted metabolites can be compared, once adjusted for a specific gravity of 1.020:

$$\text{Concentration}_{1.020} = \frac{\text{Concentration measured} \times (\text{sample specific gravity} - 1)}{(1.020 - 1)}$$

In the vast majority of male athletes' samples, the normalised concentration of testosterone and epitestosterone glucuroconjugated does not exceed 130 ng/mL, while levels lower than 30 to 40 ng/mL, often of just a few nanograms per milliliter, are measured in females' samples.[39,40] For that reason, the T/E is often given as the direct ratio of the always measurable peak area (*m/z* 432) instead of the ratio of concentrations, which cannot always be reliably quantified, particularly following the administration of testosterone. The T/E values follow a bimodal distribution that parallels the pattern found for testosterone. We observe the presence of a minor population of ratios at values below 1 due to lower excreted concentrations of testosterone glucuronide; that pattern was shown to correlate strongly with UGT2B17 (uridine diphosphoglucuronosyl transferase) deletion polymorphism, more frequent in Asians.[41]

7 Stability of individual parameters

Longitudinal studies of individual parameters collected from previous or subsequent test results, knowing the population reference ranges and their expected individual stability, could give conclusive evidence of the adminis- tration of a prohibited steroid when a value is found to be a statistical outlier to the athlete's norm.

The ratios of 5α- to 5β-metabolites (e.g. androsterone to etiocholanolone) are the most stable parameters of the individual steroid profile.[39] Generally, the T/E values of a given male individual are found to be within 30 percent of the individual mean, whether that mean is located at 1 or 6, while in females, larger variations of up to 65 percent are reported. Obviously, a disrupted profile of T/E values and concentration of testosterone glucuronide, both increased to abnormal values, reflects the administration of a prohibited steroid (Figure 4.7).

The T/E values of female volunteers and athletes show more variation: totally random fluctuations of 10 percent to 64 percent from the mean are recorded over the menstrual cycle of female volunteers, while the ratios of female athletes' samples vary to the same extent when followed over years. Nonetheless, abnor- mal fluctuations can still be picked up, as shown by the case reported in Figure 4.8, showing abnormal fluctuations of T/E values (132 percent) due to an outlier sample also found to contain higher levels of testosterone.

8 Alterations of steroid profiles by "natural" AAS

The evaluation of T/E values does not in itself allow the detection of the administration of all testosterone-related AAS. For example, dihydrotestos- terone (DHT), the 5α-reduced metabolite, produces an increased excretion of the related 5α- metabolites; it does not alter the T/E values but instead enhances the ratio of androsterone to etiocholanolone. Several adverse analytical find- ings were reported in the early 1990s, and these have apparently stopped the use of DHT as a doping agent.[42] That episode has, however, stressed the impor- tance of monitoring other parameters of the steroid profile apart from the T/E value and the concentration of testosterone and epitestosterone.

The oral administration of DHEA and androstenedione, biological precur- sors of testosterone, will not necessarily result in the increased excretion of testosterone or epitestosterone glucuronide. As a matter of fact, the ratios are not always altered, and when they are, the effects are very short-lived.[32,40,43] Marked individual variations are observed. With both steroids, the excretion of androsterone, etiocholanolone and the androstandiols is drastically increased in the following hours, but at different rates, varying with time, particularly

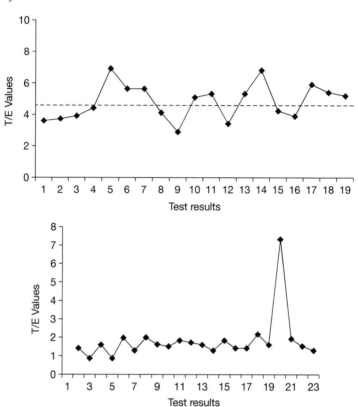

Figure 4.7 Typical variation over several years of a male athlete's 19 T/E values (dotted line for mean at 4.8 (23 percent)) (upper graph) and disrupted six-year profile of 22 T/E values in an adverse analytical finding (abnormal T/E at 7.3) (lower graph).

when DHEA is involved. While abnormal levels of DHEA glucuronide can be measured for a period of several hours, the presence of characteristic metabolites such as 6α-hydroxyandrostenedione, 6β-hydroxyepiandrosterone (sulphoconjuguated, persistent),[43] 3α,5-cyclo-5α-androstan-6β-ol-17-one[44] or the abnormal ratio of the sulphates of 7β-hydroxydehydroepiandrosterone to 16α-hydroxyandrosterone is of diagnostic value.[43] The complementary IRMS analysis is particularly useful in such cases, since the $\delta^{13}C$ values of one or two persistent metabolites still reflect their exogenous origin even when their levels are back to normal; that is, within the population reference ranges.

9 Factors influencing the steroid profile

Several supplements are advertised as having the potential to increase the natural secretion of testosterone, but those claims remain mostly unsupported. After weeks of treatment, the plant *Tribulus terrestris* had no influence on serum testosterone, androstenedione, LH or on T/E values.[45,46]

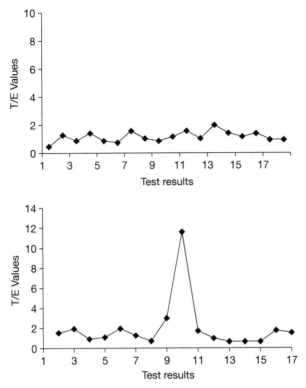

Figure 4.8 Typical variation over eight years of a female athlete's 18 T/E values (mean at 1.1 (31 percent)) (upper graph) and disrupted five-year profile of 16 T/E values in an adverse analytical finding (abnormal T/E at 11/6; mean at 2.0 (13.2 percent)) (lower graph).

Urine samples are not collected under sterile conditions, and under favorable conditions microbial growth alters the steroid profile through the hydrolysis of the conjugates and subsequent oxidation reductions leading to the disappearance of the metabolites and the accumulation of 5α- and 5β-androstan-3, 17-dione in the matrix. It is worth mentioning that neither testosterone nor any other prohibited steroids are formed during these processes, and nor do they have any influence on the $\delta^{13}C$ values of metabolites.[47,48] Finasteride, a prohibited inhibitor of the 5α-reductase, has a marked effect on the steroid profile, altering the ratios of the 5α- to 5β-metabolites (the ratio of androsterone to etiocholanolone typically goes from 1 to 0.2).[49]

Finally, the determination of the origin of urinary metabolites is essential in the most complex although very rare cases where the excretion of testosterone and T/E is drastically increased to clearly abnormal levels, by the ingestion of large, inebriating quantities of alcohol.[50] The $\delta^{13}C$ values of all the metabolites accurately reflect their endogenous origin; the confirmed presence of ethanol in the specimens confirms the "physiological condition."

10 False "negatives"

The accurate quantification of all the parameters of the steroid profile is essential to the detection of testosterone-related AAS and to permit individual follow-up. On the other hand, for the extensive purification of a relatively high volume of sample for analytes present at low levels, high levels of technical skill are required to obtain accurate results from the GC/C/IRMS analysis, and that has limited its successful implementation in all laboratories. Nonetheless, the limits of a method strictly based upon the comparison to population-based reference ranges become obvious when one considers that (1) the T/E value or concentrations of metabolites may not be increased or modified systematically, or sufficiently to exceed the range of values measured in humans if the reference population was not properly chosen;[35] (2) the alteration of T/E values following the repeated daily oral administration of testosterone is perceptible for a few hours only and is without impact on LH and epitestosterone;[51] and (3) new formulations, gels and transdermal patches, deliver testosterone in low amounts, inducing subtle modifications of the steroid profile while the results of the IRMS analysis indicate only a minor influence on androsterone and etiocholanolone, considered to be weak markers.[52]

Only the comparison of individual values would permit the systematic spotting of the effects of a testosterone-related AAS, even when injections of testosterone were involved. The expression of UGT2B17 (uridine diphospho-glucuronosyl transferase) deletion polymorphism, more frequent in certain populations, produces T/E values that are clearly lower than 1 and will remain within the population-based reference ranges – that is, under 4 – following the administration of the AAS.[35,40]

11 Conclusion

As long as the samples are collected all through the year and not only during competition, purely synthetic AAS can be detected by means of a proper selection of persistent markers and sensitive analytical methods. The situation is more problematic when natural AAS are involved, even when several parameters of the steroid profiles are monitored, since only the samples with values exceeding the norm of the reference population would be further investigated by IRMS. The identity of the athlete is blind to the laboratory, and consequently only the testing authorities can verify the individual stability of the steroid profile. With the proper statistical tools and a rapid exchange of information, the IRMS analysis could be done on a sample that upon first screening had not revealed values exceeding the population-based threshold. The measure of the $\delta^{13}C$ values of the main urinary metabolites, androsterone and etiocholanolone, is insufficient and must be extended to testosterone, DHEA and the 5α- and 5β-androstandiols.

12 References

1 Brooks RV, Firth RG, Sumner NA. Detection of anabolic steroids by radioimmunoassay. *British Journal of Sports Medicine.* 1975; 9(2): 89–92.

2 Rogozkin VA, Morozov VI, Tchaikovsky VS. Rapid radioimmunoassay for anabolic steroids in urine. *Schweizerische Zeitschrift für Sportmedizin.* 1979; 27(4): 169–73.

3 Massé R, Ayotte C, Bi HG, Dugal R. Studies on anabolic steroids. III. Detection and characterisation of stanozolol urinary metabolites in humans by gas chromatography-mass spectrometry. *Journal of Chromatography.* 1989; 497: 17–37.

4 Massé R and Goudreault D. Studies on anabolic steroids-II. 18-hydroxylated metabolites of mesterolone, methenolone and stenbolone: new steroids isolated from human urine, *J Steroid Biochm Molec Biol.* 1992; 42 (3/4): 399–410.

5 Schänzer W, Opfermann G, Donike M. Metabolism of stanozolol: identification and synthesis of urinary metabolites. *Journal of Steroid Biochemistry.* 1990; 36(1–2): 153–74.

6 Schänzer W, Delahaut P, Geyer H, Machnik M, Horning S. Long-term detection and identification of metandienone and stanozolol abuse in athletes by gas chromatography-high-resolution mass spectrometry. *Journal of Chromatography B: Analytical Techniques in the Biomedical and Life Sciences.* 1996; 687(1): 93–108.

7 Schänzer W. Metabolism of anabolic androgenic steroids. *Clinical Chemistry.* 1996; 42(7): 1001–20.

8 Schänzer W, Geyer H, Fussholler G, Halatcheva N, Kohler M, Parr MK, Guddat S, Thomas A, Thevis M. Mass spectrometric identification and characterisation of a new long-term metabolite of metandienone in human urine, *Rapid Communications in Mass Spectrometry.* 2006; 20: 2252–8.

9 Kuuranne T, Vahermo M, Leinonen A, Kostianen R. Electrospray and atmospheric pressure chemical ionization tandem mass spectrometric behavior of eight anabolic steroid glucuronides, *J Am Soc Mass Spectrom.* 2000; 11(8): 722–30.

10 Leinonen A, Kuuranne T, Kostiainen R. Liquid chromatography/mass spectrometry in anabolic steroid analysis: optimization and comparison of three ionization techniques: electrospray ionization, atmospheric pressure chemical ionization and atmospheric pressure photoionization. *Journal of Mass Spectrometry.* 2002; 37(7): 693–8.

11 Thevis M, Schänzer W. Mass spectrometry in sports drug testing: structure characterisation and analytical assays. *Mass Spectrometry Reviews.* 2007; 26: 79–107.

12 Ayotte C. Significance of 19-norandrosterone findings in athletes' urine samples. *British Journal of Sports Medicine.* 2006; 40(Suppl. 1), 25–9.

13 Massé R, Bi H, Ayotte C, Du P, Gélinas H, Dugal R. Studies on anabolic steroids V. Sequential reduction of methandienone and structurally related steroid A-ring substituents in humans: gas chromatographic-mass spectrometric study of the corresponding urinary metabolites. *Journal of Chromatography B: Analytical Techniques in the Biomedical and Life Sciences.* 1991; 562: 323–40.

14 Schänzer W, Geyer H, Donike M. Metabolism of metandienone in man: identification and synthesis of conjugated excreted urinary metabolites, determination of excretion rates and gas chromatographic-mass spectrometric identification of bishydroxylated metabolites. *Journal of Steroid Biochemistry and Molecular Biology.* 1991; 38(4): 441–64.

15 Bi H, Massé R, Just G. Studies on anabolic steroids 9. Tertiary sulfates of anabolic 17 alpha-methyl steroids: synthesis and rearrangement. *Steroids.* 1992; 57(7): 306–12.

16 Bi H, Massé R. Studies on anabolic steroids 12. Epimerization and degradation of anabolic 17 beta-sulfate-17 alpha-methyl steroids in human: qualitative and quantitative GC/MS analysis. *Journal of Steroid Biochemistry and Molecular Biology.* 1992; 42(5): 533–46.

17 Schänzer W, Opfermann G, Donike M. 17-Epimerization of 17 alpha-methyl anabolic steroids in humans: metabolism and synthesis of alpha-hydroxy-17 beta-methyl steroids. *Steroids.* 1992; 57(11): 537–40.

18 Ayotte C, Goudreault D. The detection of new synthetic drugs in athletes' urine samples. *Journal of Toxicology: Toxin Reviews*, Special Issue on Doping in Sports, Current Issues. 1999; 18(2): 113–23.

19 Bommerich U, Opfermann G, Schänzer W. Characterisation of chemically modified steroids for doping control purposes by electrospray ionisation tandem mass spectrometry. *Journal of Mass Spectrometry.* 2005; 40: 494–502.

20 Catlin DH, Ahrens BD, Kucherova Y. Detection of norbolethone, an anabolic steroid never marketed, in athletes' urine. *Rapid Communications in Mass Spectrometry.* 2002; 16(13): 1273–5.

21 Catlin DH, Sekera MH, Ahrens BD, Starcevic B, Chang Y, Hatton CK. Tetrahydrogestrinone: discovery, synthesis, and detection in urine. *Rapid Communications in Mass Spectrometry.* 2004; 18(12): 1245–9.

22 Labrie F, Luu-The V, Calvo F, Martel C, Cloutier J, Gauthier S, Belleau P, Morissette J, Lévesque MH, Labrie C. 'Tetrahydrogestrinone induces a genomic signature typical of a potent anabolic steroid. *Journal of Endocrinology*, 2005; 184: 427–33.

23 Friedel A, Geyer H, Kamber M, Laudenbach-Leschowsky U, Schänzer W, Thevis M, Vollmer G, Zierau O, Diel P. Tetrahydrogestrinone is a potent but unselective binding steroid and affects glucocorticoid signalling in the liver. *Toxicology Letters.* 2006; 164(1): 16–23.

24 Ayotte C, Goudreault D, Cyr D, Gauthier J, Ayotte P, Larochelle C, Poirier D. Characterisation of chemical and hormonal properties of new steroids related to doping of athletes, in *Proceedings of the Manfred Donike Workshop, 24th Cologne Workshop on Dope Analysis*, Cologne. 2006; 151.

25 Cross AD, Edwards JA, Orr JC, Berköz B, Cervantes L, Calzada MC, Bowers A. Steroids. CCVI. Ring A modified hormone analogs. II. 2-Methylene androstanes and 2-methyl-Δ^1, Δ^2 and Δ^3-androstenes. *Journal of Medicinal Chemistry.* 1963 March; 6: 162–6.

26 Counsell, RE, Adelstein GW, Klimstra PD, Smith B. "Anabolic agents: 19-nor- and 19-substituted 5α-androst-2-ene derivatives", *Journal of Medicinal Chemistry.* 1966; 9: 685–9.

27 Lévesque JF, Gaudreault M, Houle R, Chauret N. Evaluation of human hepatocyte incubation as a new tool for metabolism study of androstenedione and norandrostenedione in a doping control perspective. *Journal of Chromatography B: Analytical Technologies in the Biomedical and Life Sciences.* 2002; 780(1): 145–53.

28 Lévesque JF, Gaudreault M, Aubin Y, Chauret N. Discovery, biosynthesis, and structure elucidation of new metabolites of norandrostenedione using in vitro systems. *Steroids.* 2005; 70(4): 305–17.

29 Lévesque, JF, Templeton E, Trimble L, Berthelette C, Chauret N. Discovery, biosynthesis, and structure elucidation of metabolites of a doping agent and a

direct analogue, tetrahydrogestrinone and gestrinone, using human hepatocytes. *Analytical Chemistry*. 2005; 77(10): 3164–72.

30 Kuuranne T, Leinonen A, Thevis M, Schänzer W, Pystynen KH, Kostiainen R. Metabolism of "new" anabolic steroids: development of in vitro methodology in metabolite production and analytical techniques, in *Proceedings of the Manfred Donike Workshop 24th Cologne Workshop on Dope Analysis*; Sportverlag, Ed. Cologne. 2006; 161–7.

31 Donike M, Barwald KR, Klostermann K, Schanzer W, Zimmermann J. Nachweis von exogenem Testosteron in Sport. In Heck H, Hollmann W, Liesen H, Rost R, eds. *Leistung und Gesundheit*. Cologne: Deutscher Ärzte-Verlag, 1983; 293.

32 Ayotte C, Lévesque JF, Cléroux M, Lajeunesse A, Goudreault D, Fakirian A. Sport Nutritional Supplements: Quality and Doping Controls. *Canadian Journal of Applied Physiology*. 2001; 26(Suppl.): S120–S129.

33 Becchi M, Aguilera R, Farizon Y, Flament MM, Casabianca H, James P. Gas chromatography/combustion/isotope-ratio mass spectrometry analysis of urinary steroids to detect misuse of testosterone in sport. *Rapid Communications in Mass Spectrometry*. 1994; 8: 304–8.

34 Aguilera R, Becchi M, Casabianca H, Hatton CK, Catlin DH, Starcevic B, Pope HG. Improved method of detection of testosterone abuse by gas chromatography/combustion/isotope ratio mass spectrometry analysis of urinary steroids. *Journal of Mass Spectrometry*. 1996; 31: 169–76.

35 Shackleton CHL, Phillips A, Chang T, Li Y. Confirming testosterone administration by isotope ratio mass spectrometric analysis of urinary androstanediols. *Steroids*. 1997; 62(4): 379–87.

36 Shackleton CHL, Roitman E, Phillips A, Chang T. Androstanediol and 5-androstenediol profiling for detecting exogenously administered dihydrotestosterone, epitestosterone, and dehydroepiandrosterone: potential use in gas chromatography isotope ratio mass spectrometry. *Steroids*. 1997; 62(10): 665–73.

37 Horning S, Geyer H, Machnik M, Schänzer W, Hilkert A, Oebelmann, J. Detection of exogenous testosterone by 13C/12C , in *Recent Advances in Doping Analysis (4), Proceedings of the Manfred Donike Workshop on Dope Analysis*, W Schänzer, H Geyer, A Gotzmann, U Mareck-Engelke, eds. Sport und Buch Strauss Edition Sport, Koln. 1997; 275.

38 World Anti-Doping Agency. International Standard of Laboratories, TD2004EAAS, Reporting and evaluation guidance for testosterone, epitestosterone, T/E ratio and other endogenous steroids. 2004. Available from www.wada-ama.org.

39 Geyer H, Mareck-Engelke U, Schänzer W, Donike M. The Cologne protocol to follow up high testosterone/epitestosterone ratios. In: Donike M, Geyer H, Gotzmann A, Mareck-Engelke U, eds. 1996 *Recent advances in doping analysis (4), Proceedings of the Fourteenth Cologne Workshop on Dope Analysis*. Cologne: Verlag Sport und Buch Strauβ, Edition Sport, 1997; 139.

40 Lévesque JF, Ayotte C. Criteria for the detection of Androstenedione oral administration, in *Recent Advances in Doping Analysis (7), Proceedings of the 17th Cologne Workshop on Dope Analysis*, W Schänzer, H Geyer, A Gotzmann, U Mareck-Engelke, eds. Sport and Buch Straub, Köln. 1999; 169.

41 Jakobsson J, Ekström L, Inotsume N, Garle M, Lorentzon M, Ohlsson C, Roh HK, Carlström K, Rane A. Large differences in testosterone excretion in Korean and Swedish men are strongly associated with a UDP-glucuronosyl transferase

2B17 polymorphism. *Journal of Clinical Endocrinology and Metabolism.* 2006; 91(2): 687–93.

42 Donike M, Ueki M, Kuroda Y, Geyer H, Nolteernsting E, Rauth S, Schänzer W, Schindler U, Volker E, Fujisaki M. Detection of dihydrotestosterone (DHT) doping: alterations in the steroid profile and reference ranges for DHT and its 5 alpha-metabolites. *Journal of Sports Medicine and Physical Fitness.* 1995; 35(4): 235–50.

43 Lévesque JF, Ayotte C. The oral administration of DHEA: the efficiency of steroid profiling. In: Schänzer W, Geyer H, Gotzmann A, Mareck-Engelke U, eds. *Recent advances in doping analysis (7), Proceedings of the Seventeenth Cologne Workshop on Dope Analysis.* Cologne: Sport und Buch Strauß, 1999; 213.

44 Cawley AT, Hine ER, Trout GJ, George AV, Kazlauskas R. Searching for new markers of endogenous steroid administration in athletes: "looking outside the metabolic box." *Forensic Science International.* 2004; 143(2–3): 103–14.

45 Neychev VK, Mitev VI. The aphrodisiac herb *Tribulus terrestris* does not influence the androgen production in young men. *Journal of Ethnopharmacology.* 2005; 101(1–3): 319–23.

46 Rogerson S, Riches CJ, Jennings C, Weatherby RP, Meir RA, Marshall-Gradisnik SM. The effect of five weeks of *Tribulus terrestris* supplementation on muscle strength and body composition during preseason training in elite rugby league players *Journal of Strength and Conditioning Research.* 2007; 21(2): 348–53.

47 Ayotte C, Goudreault D, Charlebois A. Testing for natural and synthetic anabolic agents in human urine. *Journal of Chromatography B: Analytical Techniques in the Biomedical and Life Sciences.* 1996; 687(1): 3–25.

48 Taylor RKR, Cawley AT, Kazlauskas R, Trout GJ, George AV. Validity of carbon isotope ratio measurements for decomposed urine samples, in *Recent Advances in Doping Analysis (12), Proceedings of the 22nd Cologne Workshop on Dope Analysis,* Schanzer W, Geyer H, Gotzmann A, Mareck U, eds. Sport & Buch, Strauss, Cologne. 2004; 491.

49 Thevis M, Geyer H, Mareck U, Flenker U, Schänzer W. Doping-control analysis of the 5[alpha]-reductase inhibitor finasteride: determination of its influence on urinary steroid profiles and detection of its major urinary metabolite. *Therapeutic Drug Monitoring.* 29(2): 236–47.

50 Karila T, Kosunen V, Leinonen A, Tähtelä R, Seppälä T. High doses of alcohol increase urinary testosterone-to-epitestosterone ratio in females. *Journal of Chromatography B: Analytical Techniques in the Biomedical and Life Sciences.* 1996; 687(1): 109–16.

51 Wright F, Lafarge JP, Antréassian J, Lagoguey M, Péres G. Long term study of steroid and peptidic hormones in the plasma of healthy young men under controlled testosterone undecanoate therapy. In Hemmersbach P, Birkaland KI, eds. *Blood samples in doping control, Second International Symposium on Drugs in Sports,* Lillehammer, Norway, August 29–31, 1993. Oslo: Pensumtjeneste, 1994; 65.

52 Geyer H, Flenker U, Mareck U, Sommer F, Schänzer W. Preliminary results regarding the detection of the misuse of testosterone gel, in *Recent Advances in Doping Analysis (12).* W Schänzer, H Geyer, A Gotzmann and U Mareck (eds.) Sport und Buch Strauss, Cologne. 2004; 121–7.

5   The art of ferreting out a designer steroid

Larry D Bowers

1 Detection of "designer" steroids

Doping control testing has two distinct objectives: deterrence for the majority of athletes, and detection for the small minority of athletes who choose to cheat. Deterrence is achieved when the testing frequency, timing and menu are such that athletes choose not to use prohibited substances. Testing for deterrence must occur frequently enough to cause concern about being caught and at the same time reassure the athlete that none of their competitors can be using prohibited substances to achieve a competitive advantage. If athletes recognize either that a substance cannot be detected or that the collection process is predictable or can be manipulated, the choice not to use relies more heavily on moral reasoning and peer support for not using a prohibited substance. Given the financial and other rewards of modern sport, some would consider a process that relies on the latter premises to deter doping naïve.

Detection, particularly of "designer" drugs, requires the use of sample collection frequency and timing strategies and testing capability that are fit for purpose. This in turn requires that at least some of the characteristics of the abused substance, such as the detection window, are known or at least hypothesized. Targeted testing guided by either suspicious laboratory findings or other non-analytical information is an important element of increasing the efficiency of testing.

As was mentioned in Chapter 2, by Larry D Bowers, the WADA List of Prohibited Substances is an "open" list, meaning that substances that have similar structure and/or pharmacological activity to those examples on the List are also prohibited even though their names do not appear in the international standard. The global nature of Olympic sport is such that the pharmacopeias of many countries must be considered in developing a testing strategy. For example, a metabolite of the stimulant bromantan, which originated in Russia, was found in the urine of several athletes at the 1996 Atlanta Olympic Games. Very little scientific literature was available on the substance, and the existing Russian literature was unavailable to the Court of Arbitration for Sport (CAS) panel during the expedited hearing, owing to "holidays" in that country. From the information available, the panel was unable to conclude that bromantan was a "related substance" under the rules in effect at that time, and the athletes were exonerated.

The scientific basis for establishing that a substance is "related" is either its chemical structure or its pharmacological activity or both. The evidence can be garnered from the published scientific literature, as was the case for the stimulant modafinil, or from scientific studies. In general, CAS panels have relied on publication of scientific work in the literature to establish peer review. Within the scientific community, however, there are other means of peer review. The development of the scientific evidence in support of the "designer steroid" THG is an interesting example of what can be done.

2 Norbolethone

The first "designer steroid" to be identified in the urine of an athlete was norbolethone. The first indication that an undetectable steroid was being used was the observation that a urine sample produced by a female athlete contained no detectable endogenous steroids. Since this situation is not compatible with life, it was clear that something had suppressed normal steroid production. Follow-up testing on some occasions yielded normal-looking urinary steroid profiles and on other occasions replicated the initial unusual finding. Eventually, norbolethone metabolites were identified in the urine.[1]

A group from Wyeth Pharmaceuticals had reported norbolethone in the steroid literature in the early 1950s. Norbolethone was developed in part because the presence of an ethyl group at position 13 of the steroid ring was shown to be more anabolic than steroids with the natural methyl group at that position. Wyeth carried out a clinical trial in Canada, but never brought the drug to market. Discussions with the principal investigators convinced USADA that the source of the steroid was not from Wyeth-archived material. It was clear at that point that someone was obtaining ideas for anabolic steroids from the 1950s literaure and was not concerned about the lack of toxicity data before giving the drugs to humans.

3 Tetrahydrogestrinone

The discovery of tetrahydrogestrinone (THG) was an additional confirmation that athletes and unethical support team members were actively involved in using substances designed to avoid detection. The scientific investigation of THG began on June 4, 2003 with receipt of a phone call inquiring as to what USADA would do if it obtained evidence of doping. A "used" 1 mL insulin syringe was received on June 6. The luer tip of the syringe contained about 100 µL of a straw-colored liquid – the drop of liquid that formed the basis of an investigation that resulted in five athletes being suspended after finding the designer steroid THG in their urines. Recognizing the importance of accumulating data to prove that the substance was a "related substance" on the List, a coordinated program of scientific inquiry was initiated and coordinated by

USADA (see Table 5.1). A portion of the contents of the syringe was sent to the UCLA Olympic Analytical Laboratory with the goal of identifying the contents.

Over the course of the next two weeks, scientists at the Olympic Analytical Laboratory used high-resolution mass spectrometry, gas and liquid chromatography coupled with mass spectrometry, and various derivatization approaches to identify the compound. The molecular formula obtained from the high-resolution mass spectrometer made it clear that there were multiple double bonds in the structure. Basic knowledge of steroid chemistry and comparisons to the mass spectrum of trenbolone strongly suggested a conjugated system of three double bonds along the backbone of the steroid. As was discussed in Chapter 4, by Christiane Ayotte, knowledge of the fragmentation patterns of steroids provides information about the structure. The chemical structure of the cyclopentane D ring and its substituents indicated that the unknown compound was a synthetic steroid with an ethyl group substituted at position 13 for the methyl group of natural steroids. In addition, there was an ethyl group at the 17 position. Oximation verified that there was a keto group at the 3 position of the A ring. By mid-June, the structure of the "designer steroid" had been tentatively identified as 18a-homo-17α-ethyl-17β-hydroxy-pregna-4,9,11-trien-3-one. This structure was closely related to another prohibited steroid – gestrinone. The only structural difference was

Table 5.1 THG scientific timeline

June 6, 2003	Syringe provided to the United States Doping Agency
June 12, 2003	Portion of the contents of the luer tip provided to UCLA Olympic Analytical Laboratory (OAL)
June 16, 2003	OAL verifies that material in the syringe is a substance that has many characteristics of a previously unidentified anabolic steroid
June 19–21, 2003	US Track and Field National Championships
June 24, 2003	OAL establishes the structure of the substance from the syringe using primarily mass spectrometric techniques
July 14, 2003	OAL successfully synthesizes the compound in the syringe by reduction of gestrinone
August 13, 2003	NARL synthesizes about 100 mg of THG (in consultation with OAL); certifies reference material
August 21, 2003	THG given to primates at Southwest Foundation for Biomedical Research
September 2003	Urine from baboons analyzed by OAL
September 10, 2003	NMR results from OAL interpreted by Tom Hoye; detailed structure of THG verified
September 23, 2003	THG detected in five urine samples from the US Track and Field National Championships
October 24, 2003	NARL certifies a second preparation of 250 mg of THG
October 31, 2003	USADA provides THG reference material to all WADA-accredited laboratories
January 2004	Bioassay report from Terry Brown of Johns Hopkins University
March 2004	Initial arbitration case involving THG

the presence of a 17α-ethynyl group in gestrinone rather than the 17α-ethyl group in the "designer" steroid.

Because of the structural similarity to gestrinone, the Olympic Analytical Laboratory was able to synthesize a small amount of the designer steroid by catalytic hydrogenation of the ethynyl group of gestrinone. The product had the same chromatographic retention behavior and mass spectra as the material in the syringe. Since the synthetic material had four hydrogen atoms more than the gestrinone starting material, the scientists at the Olympic Analytical Laboratory named the "designer" steroid tetrahydrogestrinone (THG). The Olympic Analytical Laboratory conducted nuclear magnetic resonance experiments on the synthesized material. From the one- and two-dimensional homonuclear (proton-proton) correlation proton nuclear magnetic resonance data, Dr Thomas Hoye, Merck Professor of Chemistry at the University of Minnesota, was able to verify the three-dimensional positions of each of the 28 protons in THG. The positions of the double bonds in the molecule were also verified.

From a legal perspective, USADA deemed it important to have an entity other than the Olympic Analytical Laboratory synthesize reference material and to certify it under ISO criteria. A search for a readily available source of gestrinone located two potential sources outside of the United States. To save time, the material purchased by USADA from Apin Chemicals in the United Kingdom was delivered directly to the Australian Government Analytical Laboratories (AGAL) in Sydney, Australia. A project team headed by Dr Steven Westwood began synthesis and certification of THG in early August. The THG produced was characterized for purity by gas and liquid chromatography, and for structure using proton and carbon nuclear magnetic resonance spectroscopy and Fourier transform infrared spectroscopy. A small amount of the certified reference material was sent to the Olympic Analytical Laboratory to be used in the development of a urinary test for THG. The remainder of the reference material was sent to USADA in mid-August.

While the structure of the parent steroid had been determined, the urinary metabolites excreted after ingestion of THG were not known. In order to develop a urinary test for THG, it was critical to identify the metabolites found in the urine. During the AGAL synthesis project, USADA had contacted scientists involved in an "artificial human liver" project utilizing human hepatocytes at the University of Minnesota to study the metabolism of THG. By late July, USADA had also completed an application for administration of THG to a baboon at the Southwest Foundation for Biomedical Research in Dallas, Texas. Upon receipt of the certified reference material from AGAL, Dr Richard Hilderbrand of USADA hand-delivered the THG to Minneapolis and Dallas. While the project in Minneapolis did not pan out, urine collected from the baboon was sent to the Olympic Analytical Laboratory. Fortunately, the laboratory found that while there were metabolites of THG present in the urine, there were also significant amounts of THG itself present.[2] Thus, it was not necessary to identify synthetic pathways to produce certified reference materials for metabolites of THG for use in the analytical procedure. The AGAL group was commissioned to produce a second, larger batch of THG certified reference material.

An interesting characteristic of THG is that under the conditions used for routine GC/MS testing by the WADA-accredited laboratories, a number of isomeric derivatives were formed. This, combined with the trace concentrations found in urine, made the compound difficult to detect by the then routine methods. The Olympic Analytical Laboratory developed several analytical techniques involving either GC/HRMS or HPLC/MS/MS to improve detection capability for THG and its metabolites. The laboratory finally settled on an HPLC/MS/MS method. Urine samples collected at the 2003 US Track and Field National Championships were tested in September, and five samples were found to contain THG. In addition, samples collected out-of-competition and at the IAAF World Championships were analyzed, and one additional sample was found to contain THG.

While the chemical structure of THG had been definitively established, its pharmacological activity had not been studied. Professor Terry Brown of Johns Hopkins University was commissioned by USADA to test the pharmacological activity of THG in two cell-based bioassays of androgen activity. The kidney cell lines used in the studies do not naturally express the androgen receptor. By inserting the human androgen receptor gene and a reporter gene into the cells, they will bind androgen and produce a highly specific and sensitive biological response. THG was found to be a more potent androgen than any natural steroid and to be comparable in activity to the synthetic steroid methyltrienolone. Two other groups also studied the androgenic activity of THG, and reached similar conclusions.[3,4] All of this material was used in establishing that THG was a "related substance" at the initial arbitration hearing in the United Kingdom.

3 Desoxymethyltestosterone (DMT) or madol

An additional steroid was seized in the BALCO raid. Its identity was eventually determined by the Olympic Analytical Laboratory to be 17α-methyl-17β-hydroxy-androst-2-ene.[5] At about the same time, the Canadian Customs Service seized a vial of material at the border. The WADA-accredited laboratory in Montreal did extensive testing and characterization of the compound independently of the studies at the Olympic Analytical Laboratory. The Montreal laboratory named the compound desoxymethyltestosterone (DMT) whereas the Olympic Analytical Laboratory named it madol. DMT has also been shown to be a potent anabolic steroid.[6]

The potential availability of undetectable steroids and other performance-enhancing substances poses a difficult problem for anti-doping science. Testing methods must be frequently monitored to ensure that evidence of new substances can be detected. Increased attention to the testing history of the athlete can provide valuable information about nonphysiological changes that occur when undetectable agents are administered. Communication between the WADA-accredited laboratories, the national anti-doping agencies and international federations, and law enforcement officials is becoming more important to identify new agents. The availability of new substances on the Internet must be monitored. Educational materials must be made available to both athletes and their support personnel regarding the potential health risks associated with ingesting uncharacterized compounds. When a complete program of anti-doping activity is put in place, the clean athlete can be reassured that there is a level playing field.

4 References

1   Catlin DH, Ahrens BD, Kucherova Y. Detection of norbolethone, an anabolic steroid never marketed, in athletes' urine. *Rapid Communications in Mass Spectrometry*. 2002; 16: 1273–5.

2   Catlin DH, Sekera MH, Ahrens BD, Starcevic B, Chang YC, Hatton CK. Tetrahydrogestrinone: discovery, synthesis, and detection in urine. *Rapid Communications in Mass Spectrometry*, 2004; 18: 1245–9.

3   Death AK, McGrath KC, Kazlauskas R, Handelsman DJ. Tetrahydrogestrinone is a potent androgen and progestin. *Journal of Clinical Endocrinology and Metabolism*. 2004; 89: 2498–500.

4   Jasuja R, Catlin DH, Miller A, Chang YC, Herbst KL, Starcevic B, Artaza JN, Singh R, Datta G, Sarkissian A, Chandsawanbhuwana C, Baker M, Bhasin S. Tetrahydrogestrinone is an androgenic steroid that stimulates androgen receptor-mediated, myogenic differentiation in C3H10T1/2 multipotent mesenchymal cells and promotes muscle accretion in orchidectomized male rats. *Endocrinology*. 2005; 146: 4472–8.

5   Sekera MH, Ahrens BD, Chang YC, Starcevic B, Georgakopoulos C, Catlin DH. Another designer steroid: discovery, synthesis, and detection of "madol" in urine. *Rapid Communications in Mass Spectrometry*. 2005; 19: 781–4.

6   Diel P, Friedel A, Geyer H, Kamber M, Laudenbach-Leschowsky U, Schänzer W, Thevis M, Vollmer G, Zierau O. Characterisation of the pharmacological profile of desoxymethyltestosterone (Madol), a steroid misused for doping. *Toxicology Letters*. 2007; 28: 64–71.

6 Isotope Ratio Mass Spectrometry
Carbon isotope ratio analysis

Rodrigo Aguilera

1 Preface

William Crookes, the father of the discovery of isotopes, wrote in 1886 in the journal *Nature*:

> When we say that the atomic mass of calcium is 40, what we are trying to say is that the core part of atoms of calcium is 40, but there is a small number of atoms which have a mass 39 and 41. Others much smaller are 38 and 42 and so forth.

He was trying to say that the atomic mass measured by chemists was in fact an average of the masses of different atoms from the same element, these various masses being very close to each other.

2 Introduction

From antiquity, human beings have tried to increase their physical performance by using artificial means. The Incas since time immemorial have used coca leaves in order to endure high altitudes and long working days. The Vikings ate mushrooms containing muscarin to face bloody battles.

Historians describe practices that to us often seem strange by which athletes attempted to increase their physical force and their muscular mass. Long jumpers, for example, ate goat meat, boxers and the javelin throwers ate bull meat and wrestlers ate fatty pork. Today, unfortunately, these very imaginative and healthy dietetic practices have disappeared, leaving in their place the doping products that appeared in sport at the end of the 1950s. Since then the problem has worsened, with serious and, in certain cases, tragic consequences.

Unfortunately, the enormous progress achieved during these past years in the pharmaceutical and medical fields, as well as the imagination of those who profit and encourage the use of anabolic products, have allowed doping practices to seep into the heart of the majority of sports today. Thus, these practices not only touch high-level athletes more and more, but also extend to participants in other sports, including amateurs and young people.

Conscious of the sheer size of the problem and the health dangers involved, and knowing that these practices are in opposition to the principles of sport, which should be to promote a healthy activity with equal chances for all the participants, the International Olympic Committee (IOC) and many other international and national sporting federations have developed means of fighting against doping. The IOC has created a medical commission in charge of studying, setting up and developing the means to control doping. With regard to the use of anabolic steroids, several methods of analysis have been proposed for the detection and identification of these compounds. The method currently recognized by the IOC for steroid analysis is based upon gas chromatography/mass spectrometry. These analyses become more difficult when the analysis of endogenous steroids is involved.

In the case of the control of testosterone doping, the method currently used consists of measuring the ratio of testosterone to epitestosterone in urine. This ratio in the majority of individuals is close to 1, but in the event of doping with testosterone, it increases. According to rules of the IOC (WADA), a case can be declared positive if this ratio is equal to or greater than 4.

However, the results of this method of analysis highlight some problems, because in certain cases the ratio is naturally greater than 4 without doping, sometimes because of physiological and pathological conditions. In addition, values of T/E ranging between 2 and 4 are not deemed to be suspicious, and are not causes for investigation of cases where the subject is in the process of eliminating the exogenous testosterone or has taken testosterone and epitestosterone simultaneously.

Because of this ambiguity, a new approach of measurement has been developed, isotopic ratio mass spectrometry based on the analysis of carbon. This technique had already been used in other fields, especially in agricultural monitoring, where it is used for detecting fraudulent products. It permits the differentiation of endogenous testosterone biosynthesized by humans from synthetic or pharmaceutical exogenous testosterone used as a doping agent.

The aim of this chapter is to explain the basic concepts of the isotope ratio mass spectrometry technique such as the fundamental notion of isotopes, and the instrumentation, applications and methodology used to differentiate endogenous from exogenous steroids. In order to make clear the principles of this technique, a basic and simple definition will be given for each part of the isotope/ratio/mass/spectrometry/carbon/analysis.

3 Definition of "atom"

In chemistry and physics, an atom (from the Greek *átomos*, meaning "the smallest indivisible particle of matter, i.e. something that cannot be divided") is the smallest particle that still characterizes a chemical element.[1] An atom consists of a dense nucleus of positively charged particles named protons and electrically neutral particles named neutrons, surrounded by a much larger electron cloud consisting of negatively charged electrons. Therefore, an atom

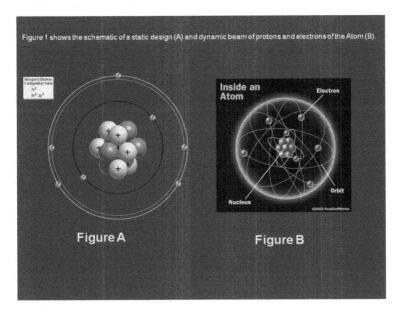

Figure 6.1 Schematic of a static design (A) and dynamic beam of protons and electrons of the atom (B).

is electrically neutral because it has the same number of protons as electrons. The number of protons in an atom defines the chemical element to which it belongs, whereas the number of neutrons determines the isotope of the element, as will become clear.

4 Definition of "isotope"

In order to define the concept of an isotope, it is important to know that the atomic mass (A) of an atom is defined by the weight of the number of protons and neutrons in its nucleus. The electrons are not taken into account, as we know that their mass is 2,000 times less than that of protons.[2] Atoms are very light in weight; one oxygen atom weighs only 0.000000000000000000000027 g. Because such a number is impractical to use, chemists instead use a unit based on an atomic standard of reference, carbon of mass 12, which is written ^{12}C. Another concept about an atom is the atomic number, which corresponds to the number of protons (which is equal to the number of electrons), namely Z.[3]

Because the atomic mass is determined by the sum of the number of protons and neutrons contained in the nucleus, two atoms of, say, carbon that have a different number of neutrons, hence a different mass, are referred to as different isotopes of carbon. For example, carbon-12 and carbon-13 are referred to as different isotopes because ^{13}C has one extra neutron in the nucleus. Since they contain the same number of protons (and hence electrons), isotopes have the same chemical properties. However, the nuclear and atomic properties of isotopes can be different. The electronic energy levels of an atom depend upon the nuclear mass. Thus, corresponding atomic levels of isotopes are slightly shifted relative to each other.

Since the construction of the Periodic Table of the Elements, initiated by Mendeleyev, over 120 elements have been confirmed so far. Of these, 81 have at least one stable isotope, whereas the rest exist only in the form of radio active nuclides. Some radioactive nuclides (e.g. ^{115}In, ^{232}Th, ^{235}U, ^{238}U) have survived from the time the elements were formed. Several thousand radioactive nuclides produced through natural or artificial means have been also identified.

Of the 83 elements that occur naturally in significant quantities on Earth, 20 are found as single isotopes (and are referred to as mononuclidic), and the others occur as admixtures containing from two to ten isotopes.[4] In IUPAC (the International Union of Pure and Applied Chemistry) nomenclature, isotopes and nuclides are specified by the name of the element, implicitly giving the atomic number, which is always the same for any particular element, followed by a hyphen and the mass number (e.g. helium-3, carbon-12, carbon-13, iodine-131, uranium-238). In symbolic form, the number of nucleons is denoted as a superscript prefix to the chemical symbol (e.g. ^{3}He, ^{12}C, ^{13}C, ^{131}I, ^{238}U).

5 Molecular mass of isotopes

The molecular mass (M_r) of an element is determined by its nucleons. For example, carbon-12 (^{12}C) has six protons and six neutrons. When a sample contains two isotopes, the equation below is applied, where M_r (1) and M_r (2) are the molecular masses of each individual isotope, and % abundance is the percentage abundance of that isotope in the sample.[1]

$$M_r = \frac{M_r(1) \times \% \text{ abundance} + M_r(2) \times \% \text{ abundance}}{100}$$

6 Mass spectrometry

Mass spectrometry is an analytical technique that is used to determine the masses of atoms or molecules in which an electrical charge is placed on the molecule and the resulting ions are separated by their mass to charge ratio. To analyze a molecule or atom by this method, we have to put them in the gas phase, and so the species must be ionized, formed into a beam, accelerated by an electric field, deflected in a magnetic or electric field, and finally detected. All these processes take place in a mass spectrometer (Figure 6.2), which consists of three separate sections: the source (ionization process), the mass analyzer (mass separation according to the mass:charge ratio) and the collector (detection).[5]

Nowadays, different technologies have been implemented to perform all kind of analysis using mass spectrometry from elemental composition to the

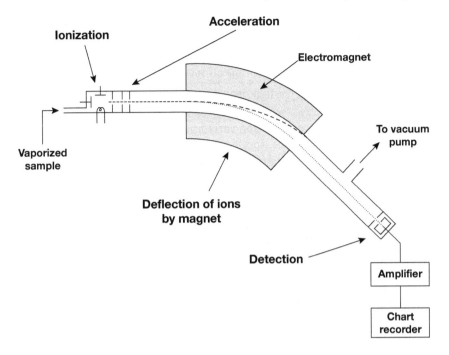

Figure 6.2 Schematic diagram of a mass spectrometer.

fields of proteomics and metabolomics. However, it is outside the scope of this chapter to cover all the instruments or technologies; hence, a specific description will be restricted to isotope ratio mass spectrometry instrumentation. Nonetheless, in order to establish some criteria concerning this instrument, and a description of it, one crucial topic has to be dealt with before we examine this technique in more depth. That topic is photosynthesis and other natural cyclic processes.

7 Review of the notion of isotopes

Atoms constituting organic matter generally exist in various isotopic forms, as described previously. The two stable isotopes of carbon, ^{12}C and ^{13}C, are the principal components of the majority of live or fossil biological entities, natural organic molecules or synthetic ones. Of these, ^{12}C is the prevalent isotope since its natural relative abundance is 98.9 percent whereas ^{13}C represents only 1.1 percent. Nonetheless, this natural abundance of isotopes is not a fixed constant; it can demonstrate significant variation, with the proportion of ^{13}C atoms sometimes being as low as 0.1 percent. The isotopic distribution of a molecule can be obtained with a high degree of accuracy and precision by isotope ratio mass spectrometry (IRMS). Indeed, this tool makes it possible to determine the isotope ratio (R) or isotope abundance (A):[6]

$$R = \frac{\text{Number of isotope atoms}}{\text{Number of light isotope atoms}}$$

$$A = \frac{\text{Number of heavy isotope atoms}}{\text{Number of heavy + light isotope atoms}}$$

Because the natural isotopic carbon variations are relatively weak (about 0.03 percent for plants), a notation specific to IRMS is used to exploit the results. The isotopic values of ratios are given compared with an international reference, and the results are expressed in delta per mille ($\delta^{13}C‰$).[7] Originally this reference was the PDB (Pee Dee Belemnite), calcium carbonate rich in ^{13}C (1.1237199 percent of isotope ^{13}C), but as stocks of PDB started to be exhausted, IUPAC recommended in 1994 that the values of δ (^{13}C) were to be reported relative to VPDB (Vienna PDB), assigning a value of +1.95 percent on the VPDB scale with the material of reference of the IAEA, International Atomic Energy Agency, NBS-19 ($CaCO_3$). In 1995, the Commission on Atomic Weights and Isotopic Abundances (CAWIA), made up of experts from various countries, published a report on the definitive need to give up the use of PDB for the expression of isotopic deviations of carbon. The value for the NBS-19 relating to the VPDB was adopted by groups of experts on the standards of stable isotopes in geochemistry and hydrology. These experts, brought together by the IAEA since the mid-1980s, had recognized the lack of reference material available and expressed on a standardized scale. In 1996, Coplen published an article officially defining the VPDB as the international reference for the measurement of the isotope ratios of carbon.[3] The results are thus expressed in delta per mille compared to VPDB ($\delta_{VPDB}^{13}C$) according to the definition:

$$\delta_{VPBB}^{13}C = \frac{(R_{sample} - R_{VPBD})}{R_{VPDB}} \times 10^3$$

where R_{sample} is the ratio $^{13}C/^{12}C$ measured for a given sample, and RVPDB is the ratio $^{13}C/^{12}C$ measured for a definite standard gauge compared to the scale of the VPDB. Because the material of reference, NBS-19, is available only in small quantities, standard solutions such as mixtures of alkanes, whose values have been gauged relative to the VPDB, are used to calibrate instruments, as will be described later in the chapter.[8]

8 Photosynthesis

One of the most important processes affecting changes in the carbon isotopic composition is the geochemical cycle, which is the abstraction of carbon from the carbon dioxide reservoir in the atmosphere and surface waters by

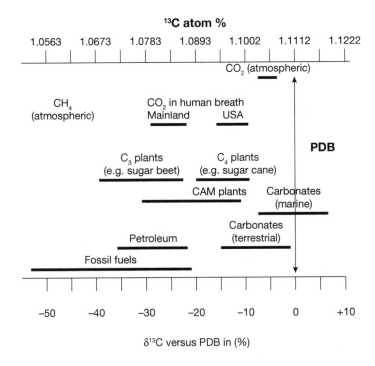

Figure 6.3 Isotope distribution in ^{13}C atom % and δ per mille versus PDB for different compounds.

photosynthetic fixation in the form of complex organic molecules. In general, such carbon shows a high degree of enrichment in the light isotope compared to its source. The products of this process are either subject to rapid decay or are incorporated into sedimentary rocks and occur there as solids, liquids or gases, either in dispersed form or concentrated, in the latter case often forming deposits of the fossil fuels, coal, petroleum or natural gases that are capable of being mined. The isotopic composition of the carbon fixed in this manner is governed by the process of photosynthesis, as well as by any subsequent changes occurring during accumulation, diagenesis, katagenesis and metamorphism, as well as migration processes.[9] In this chapter, the isotopic fractionation during photosynthesis and the isotopic composition of the resulting products will be reviewed to help make clear why carbon isotope ratio analysis has been used to differentiate synthetic from endogenous testosterone and other exogenous or endogenous steroids. Particularly important is the fact that pharmaceutical testosterone comes from hemisynthesis by plants.

Carbon fixation in photosynthesis proceeds by one of two pathways, depending on the species of plant. The pathways differ by the number of carbon atoms in the first-formed intermediate compounds. The two pathways are known as the Calvin-Benson (C_3 or non-Kranz) cycle and the Kranz (C_4)

cycle respectively. The carbon isotopic composition of the plant material formed correlates strongly with the type of photosynthetic cycle followed by the particular organism.

9 Origins of isotopic discrimination by plants

The natural abundance of ^{13}C in the carbon skeleton of molecules varies from one organism to another. These differences are due to the existence of various ways of assimilating and fixing carbon during photosynthesis. During this process, the heavy isotopes (^{13}C) and light isotopes (^{12}C) of the same element have slightly different kinetic reaction constants, a phenomenon known as natural isotopic fractionation. Thus, the molecules with a greater quantity of ^{13}C in their structure are enriched in ^{13}C, while those having a smaller quantity of ^{13}C are depleted in ^{13}C. The plants generate carbon molecules by integrating atmospheric carbon via photosynthesis. We can classify the metabolic photosynthesis of plants into three main categories: C_3-type species, C_4-type species and species of the CAM (crassulacean acid metabolism) type. Each of these species achieves the incorporation of atmospheric CO_2 via to a well-defined cycle.[10,11]

9.1 *C₃-type plants*

The cycle of photosynthetic reduction of CO_2 that takes place in plants of the C_3 type is called the Calvin–Benson cycle (Figure 6.4). This cycle includes 14 reactions that take place during the dark phase of photosynthesis. Atmospheric CO_2 is caused to react with a sugar phosphate with 5 carbon atoms, ribulose-1,5-diphosphate. The first stable product identified in this reaction is glycerate-3-phosphate, with three carbon atoms (which is where the C_3 designation comes from). The incorporation (fixation) of CO_2 is achieved by the action of the ribulose-1,5-diphosphate carboxylase by an intramolecular oxidoreduction, or dismutation reaction. This first compound, characteristic of the C_3 plants, is then transformed into various sugars via complex enzymatic reactions, eventually returning to the starting product, ribulose-1,5-diphosphate. This cycle occurs in 80–90 percent of crop plants, including wheat, rice, potatoes, soy and sugar beet.[11]

9.2 *C₄-type plants*

The cycle of photosynthetic reduction of CO_2 of plants of the C_4-type is called the Hatch–Slack cycle (Figure 6.5). In C_4-type plants, the photosynthetic reduction of CO_2 requires two successive carboxylations. The first, which takes place in the cells of the mesophyll leaves, uses external atmospheric CO_2. Under the action of the phosphoenolpyruvate carboxylase, CO_2 will be fixed on a substrate, phosphoenolpyruvate, to give oxaloacetate

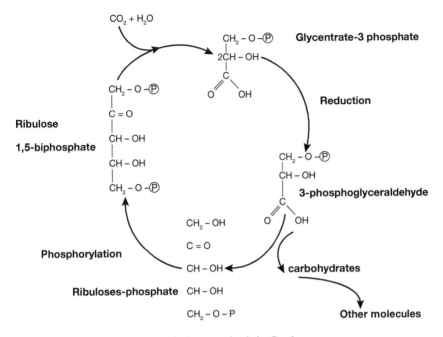

Figure 6.4 Metabolic pathway of photosynthesis in C_3 plants.

(which has four carbon atoms). This unstable compound will be converted into malate and aspartate under the action of specific enzymes, then into pyruvate and subsequently phosphoenolpyruvate. CO_2 released during these reactions is fixed once more onto ribulose-1,5-diphosphate under the action of ribulose-1,5-diphosphate carboxylase, and then reduced by the sequence of reactions of the Calvin–Benson cycle. The plants characteristic of this way of fixing CO_2 are maize, cane sugar and certain fodders.[10]

9.3 Plants of the crassulacean acid metabolism (CAM) type

The third group of plants corresponds to the Crassulaceae. These species are characterized by their double photosynthetic processes, which is a mixed combination of the Calvin–Benson and the Hatch-Slack cycles. In darkness, these plants are able to bind great quantities of CO_2, thus giving rise to a large amount of malate via phosphoenolpyruvate carboxylase. The malate thus accumulated in darkness is then decarboxylated in light under the action of malate dehydrogenase. Then the released CO_2 again reacts with ribulose-1,5-diphosphate in a reaction catalyzed by ribulose-1,5-diphosphate carboxylase and reduced by the Calvin–Benson cycle. To summarize, in this category of plants CO_2 is captured at night via the C_4 cycle, then is released into the leaves to be fixed via the C_3 cycle during the following day.[1]

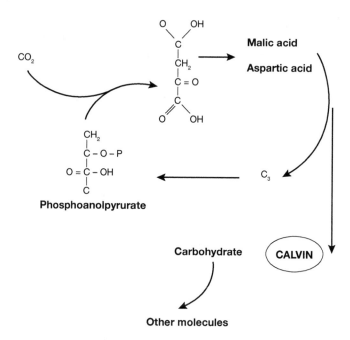

CO$_2$

Malic acid

Aspartic acid

Phosphoanolpyrurate

C$_3$

Carbohydrate

CALVIN

Other molecules

Figure 6.5 Metabolic pathway of photosynthesis in C$_4$ plants.

Even though all these plants use the Calvin–Benson cycle for the photosynthetic reduction of CO_2, differences remain. For C$_3$ plants, the carboxylation stage is irreversible. This initial reaction plays a major part in the determination of isotopic fractionation appearing in these plants. Indeed, the enzyme ribulose-1,5-diphosphate carboxylase discriminates with regard to carbon-13. The result is that, compared to C$_3$ species, C$_4$ species and, frequently but not always, CAM-type species, appear enriched in ^{13}C. Relative enrichment in ^{13}C of CAM-type plants is in fact very variable owing to the fact that, depending on the conditions, CO_2 can be bound predominantly either by phosphoenolpyruvate carboxylase or by ribulose 1,5-diphosphate carboxylase. Thus, according to the type of plant examined, the isotopic deviations obtained will be relatively enriched for C$_4$ plants and relatively impoverished for C$_3$ plants (Figure 6.4). It is this physiological difference that is at the origin of the various isotopic deviations measured for different compounds. The natural molecules resulting from these plants maintain a specific isotopic signature stemming from their environment and the types of photosynthesis.[1]

10 Isotope Ratio Mass Spectrometry

The use of steroid hormones to enhance performances by athletes has been strictly prohibited by the International Olympic Committee and other international sport organizations since the end of the 1960s. The rules are enforced, and regulate the use of these substances. However, with regard to steroid hormones that are acknowledged as being natural, there is currently no definitive method available to differentiate natural steroids from exogenous ones. Methods based on measuring the testosterone/epitestosterone ratio are contestable, taking into account inter- and intra-individual variability, including variations resulting from physiological and pathological conditions. IRMS coupled to gas chromatography–combustion (GC–C–IRMS) represents a new approach in this field, insofar as it makes it possible to determine the origin of organic substances. Numerous preliminary studies have established that this technique could in many cases reveal any exogenous administration. This section of the chapter will describe how the technique is used for the analytical measurement of steroids.

Steroid hormones are present in trace amounts in urine, blood, tissue, fecal matter, etc.[12] However, it is in urine that the concentration of steroid hormones remains most significant, at about 10–100 µg/L. In muscle, one may find concentrations of micrograms per liter or even nanograms per liter. Nevertheless, the GC–C–IRMS is a technique of limited sensitivity. In order to reliably determine the $^{13}C/^{12}C$ ratio of a molecule, concentrations of tens of micrograms per liter are necessary. Below this threshold, the limitations of the equipment are reached and measurements are no longer reliable.

Before any isotopic measurements can be taken, in the case of a matrix such as urine, multiple stages of purification and extraction of the relevant molecules are necessary. All the targeted molecules must be introduced separately one by one into the IRMS analyzer, and the interferences generated by the matrix (biological background noise) must be eliminated while minimizing the losses of analytes by these multiple stages. In order to achieve this, various liquid–liquid or solid–liquid techniques of extraction and purification have been used in analytical chemistry, but these will not be described in this chapter.

To analyze any organic or inorganic molecules by isotope ratio measurement, it is necessary to transform the molecules, by oxidation, pyrolysis or reduction, into an elementary simple gas, such as CO_2 in the case of carbon isotope analysis. The total process is carried out in an isotopic ratio mass spectrometer coupled to a gas chromatograph (GC) via a furnace (C) for the combustion of the molecules (GC–C–IRMS). Figure 6.6 is a schematic diagram showing the basic elements that constitute this equipment.[10]

The analytes traverse a well-defined pathway during which they will undergo the following processes:

•   The sample molecules are separated via the chromatographic column in the gas phase.

GC–C–IRMS INTERFACE

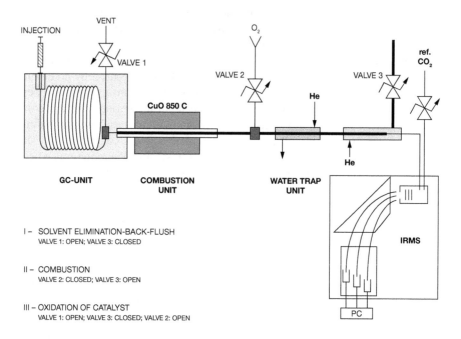

Figure 6.6 Diagram of the principal parts of an isotope ratio mass spectrometer coupled to a gas chromatograph via a combustion oven.

- The designated compounds are converted into the elementary gases CO_2 and H_2O in the combustion oven.
- The water molecules are retained in the water trap and only the molecules of CO_2 reach the source of the mass spectrometer, where they undergo ionization by electronic impact.
- The ions formed in the source are separated magnetically according to their characteristic masses; the isotopomers of CO_2 are consequently separated.
- A computer calculates the $^{13}C/^{12}C$ isotopic ratios of the analytes using the value of the isotopic ratio of the reference CO_2 introduced directly into the source and calibrated to an internationally accepted reference substance (VPDB).

11 Gas chromatography

The gas chromatograph (GC) used for coupled GC/C/IRMS is the same as the type used in simple GC/MS. The column and conditions must be the same as those used for GC/MS for it to be possible to compare the chromatograms obtained by the two instruments. In the oven of the GC, the entry of the column is connected to the split or splitless injector functioning in splitless mode. In this mode, the sample is vaporized in the injector and is concentrated at the head of column during a one-minute delay. The total volume injected is then introduced in the capillary column by the carrier gas (helium). The components of the sample are then separated according to their boiling point and their affinity for the stationary phase. By a specific device in the system, the effluent of column can be directed either towards a valve ("heart split", HS) making it possible to evacuate the undesirable compounds, or toward the mass spectrometer (via the combustion oven). A flame ionization detector (FID) can be connected as a type of valve HS to characterize the compounds before combustion if necessary.[13]

11.1 The combustion interface

The combustion interface is made up of three elements:

- A thermostat-controlled interface allows a connection between the GC oven and the module containing the furnace.
- The module containing the combustion oven is a thermostat-controlled enclosure whose temperature is regulated to 850–940 °C.
- The combustion oven is a quartz or ceramic tube. The tubing can be filled with copper oxide granules threaded one behind the other and blocked at the end of the tube by silver wool wire, or the filling can be composed of two twisted wires of platinum and copper respectively. The copper oxide possesses the property of being able to release oxygen at high temperatures (850–940 °C), which is essential to combustion. The compounds are then instantaneously burned and transformed into the simple gases CO_2 and H_2O.

11.2 The water trap

The water formed via the combustion oven must be eliminated so that no trace of water is introduced into the source of the mass spectrometer. Indeed, the smallest trace of water could lead to the protonation of the $^{12}CO_2$ to give

Table 6.1 Common elements and corresponding gases measured by IRMS

Element		Gas	Abundance	Raw material
H	$^2H/^1H$	H_2	0.015%	Water, methane, cellulose
C	$^{13}C/^{12}C$	CO_2	1.1%	CO_2, organics, carbonate
N	$^{15}N/^{14}N$	N_2	0.3%	N_2, NH_4, nitrates
O	$^{18}O/^{16}O$	CO_2, CO	0.2%	CO_2, H_2O, organics
S	$^{34}S/^{32}S$	SF_6, SO_2	4.2%	Sulfates, sulfides, organics

$H^{12}CO_2^+$, which would interfere with the measurement of $^{13}CO_2$ (isobaric interferences). There are two means of eliminating this water: the cryogenic water trap and the Nafion® membrane.

The cryogenic trap consists of a Dewar vessel (container resistant to very low temperatures) filled with liquid nitrogen, into which the water trap is plunged. This trap is composed of two twisted capillaries, one being a stainless steel capillary and the other a heating resistor. A thermostat is connected to the steel capillary so that the temperature is maintained at $-100\ °C$. At this temperature, only the CO_2 molecules will be able to cross the cooled capillary. The water molecules will be retained by the trap.[11]

The Nafion® membrane is a hydrophilic membrane that selectively absorbs the water in the gas current which is circulating. Water is expelled through the membrane by osmosis and is evacuated by circulating auxiliary gas (Helium).

11.3   The isotope ratio mass spectrometer

The source of the spectrometer is a small ionization chamber in which electrons are emitted by an incandescent filament and accelerated by the application of a potential difference. The CO_2 gas molecules are ionized to $CO_2^{+\cdot}$ by collision with the electron beam. The mode of ionization of this source is electronic impact (EI), functioning with an energy of 70 eV. When they enter the source, the electrons pass through a narrow slit and are thus focused into a beam. In the interior of the source, the flow of electrons follows a helicoid trajectory under the influence of a magnetic field produced by two small magnets placed on both sides of the source. This helicoid trajectory makes it possible to increase the probability of collision between electrons and gas molecules introduced into the source. The majority of the electrons, those that do not cause ionization, are collected on an electron trap called the "trap." The current at the trap provides feedback that makes it possible to regulate and control the emission of the filament and thereby maintain a constant flow of electrons through the source. The ions formed (m/z 44, 45, 46) are then pushed back towards the outlet of the ionization chamber by a metal lens (repeller). A system of charged lenses helps the extraction, focusing the ions in space (according to the x, y, z axes) and then accelerating them.

The mass analyzer is composed of a low-resolution magnetic sector with an asymmetrical geometry of 90 °. With this particular geometry, all the masses are separated and focused simultaneously.

The mass detector consists of several collectors of the Faraday cap type. Each of these collectors collects only one given mass. For the determination of the isotope ratios of carbon, three collectors are enough: for mass 44, for mass 45 and one for mass 46 (Figure 6.7). The currents detected in these collectors are proportional to the respective quantity of each type of ion being collected.

From Table 6.2, it is possible to deduce the ratios of these relative abundances from the abundance of the isotopic peaks obtained from the carbon dioxide analyzed (m/z 44, 45 and 46).

m/z 44: 100%

m/z 45: (1.1 + 0.04 + 0.04) = 1.18%

m/z 46: 0.2 + 0.2 + (0.04 × 0.04) + (1.1 × 0.04) + (1.1 × 0.04) = 0.49%

Stable Isotopes

^{12}C majority	^{16}O majority
^{13}C minority	^{17}O minority
	^{18}O minority

Faraday caps detection

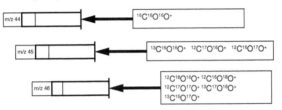

Figure 6.7 Isotopomer ions of CO_2 collected in the cages of the Faraday cap for the *m/z* ratios 44, 45 and 46. The relative abundances of the carbon and oxygen isotopes are shown in Table 6.2.

Table 6.2 Relative abundances of the isotopes of carbon and oxygen measured in steroid analysis

Isotope	Relative abundance (%)
^{12}C	100
^{13}C	1.1
^{16}O	100
^{17}O	0.04
^{18}O	0.2

Table 6.3 The different isotope ranges for organic molecules

Organic molecule	Isotope composition (δ per mille)
Animals	−15 to 25‰
C_3 plants	−22 to 40‰
C_4 plants	−8 to 20‰
Natural gas	−30 to 50‰
Coal	−25 to 30‰
Petroleum	−25 to 30‰

12 Measurement of $^{13}C/^{12}C$ ratios

The determination of $^{13}C/^{12}C$ ratios of the analytes is carried out by examining the ratio of the intensities of the signals collected for m/z 44 and 45. Mass-to-change ratio 44 corresponds to CO_2 with carbon-12 ($^{12}C^{16}O^{16}O$), while 45 corresponds to CO_2 with the carbon-13 isotope ($^{13}C^{16}O^{16}O$). However, the mass-to-change ratio 45 also corresponds to isotopomers $^{12}C^{17}O^{16}O$ or $^{12}C^{16}O^{17}O$. The signal detected in the collector of mass-to-change 45 will thus be a mixture of the signals of ion $^{13}C^{16}O^{16}O^{+\cdot}$ and of ions $^{12}C^{17}O^{16}O^{+\cdot}$ and $^{12}C^{16}O^{17}O^{+\cdot}$. Ions $^{12}C^{17}O^{16}O^{+\cdot}$ and $^{12}C^{16}O^{17}O^{+\cdot}$ coming from an isotope of oxygen present as a substantial proportion will thus interfere with the signal coming from ion $^{13}C^{16}O^{16}O^{+\cdot}$ (which has the same m/z ratio). The intensity of signal 45 could thus be distorted if no corrections are made. It is thus necessary to have an exact knowledge of the specific contribution of the ions $^{12}C^{17}O^{16}O^{+\cdot}$ and $^{12}C^{16}O^{17}O^{+\cdot}$ in order to determine the isotopic ratio $^{13}C/^{12}C$ precisely. This correction, calculated by the software, is based on the relation of Craig,[7] and relies on the signal collected for mass 46. In fact, the intensity measured at the collector or signal 46 integrates the contribution of ^{18}O and makes it possible to deduce the contribution from ^{17}O. The type of ion associating ^{13}C and ^{17}O is rare; isotopomer $^{13}C^{17}O^{16}O^{+\cdot}$ is thus not taken into account. The signal recorded for mass-to-change 46 thus provides information about the quantity of ^{17}O and ^{18}O present in CO_2 of the analytes. The formula used by the software to carry out the correction is as follows:

$$\frac{^{17}O}{^{16}O} = K\left(\frac{^{18}O}{^{16}O}\right)^a$$

where $a = 0.516$ and $K = 0.0099235$. This correction is applied by default by the software. However, another approach, described by Santrock and Hayes,[14] suggests an alternative algorithm for this correction but is not officially recognized at an international level. According to these authors, the Craig correction usually employed can generate systematic errors in the measurement of abundance in ^{13}C, and these errors would be reflected in the findings for the absolute abundance of ^{17}O. Two additional constants are needed in these calculations to avoid possible errors; they correspond to ratios $^{13}C/^{12}C$ ($^{13}R_{VPDB}$) and $^{18}O/^{16}O$ ($^{18}R_{VPDB}$). The values of these constants have been determined as follows:

$$^{13}R_{VPDB} = 0.0112372$$

$$^{18}R_{VPDB} = 0.0020079$$

These constants can be inserted in the parameters of the reprocessing software, but only by the service engineer. However, before using these constants the user must check that they are correct; if not, the final results will most likely be erroneous.

13 Introduction of reference CO_2

A reference sample of CO_2 of known $^{13}C/^{12}C$ isotope ratio, is injected several times in the form of a "pulse" in order to determine the isotopic deviation of the compounds compared to VPDB ($\delta^{13}C_{VPDB}$). The CO_2 bottle is connected to an injection system of reference gas in which a mechanical valve for airless injection is contained. This valve (valve RG) contains a silica capillary of 25 μm (i.d.) which allows the CO_2 and the current of helium to be transported towards the mass spectrometer. At the time the piston causing the entry of CO_2 is activated, by a compressed air system, this gas current will be directed toward the standby valve. This valve makes it possible to protect the mass spectrometer when the operating conditions of the apparatus are not optimal, while allowing the introduction of reference CO_2 into the source.

14 A new concept for isotope ratio mass spectrometry: IRM-LC/MS

A new interface to couple a liquid chromatograph (LC) with an isotope ratio mass spectrometer has been developed during the past few years.[15] This interface applies particularly to the determination of $^{13}C/^{12}C$ ratios in organic compounds. The first tests concerning the IRM-LC/MS coupling date from the 1990s. Osborn and Abramson[16] described a first system where the solvent resulting from the LC was vaporized in a heated area, which allows the desolvation of the sample. Caimi and Brenna[17] described an interface that allows the deposit of the fluent on a mobile belt or "moving belt"; the solvent is evaporated there and the analytes deposited before sublimation and combustion.

In these new types of interfaces, the solvent is not eliminated from the sample, which undergoes oxidation (CuO/Pt). The sample is oxidized while it is still in the mobile phase, and only afterwards is CO_2 separated from the liquid phase and analyzed in the isotope ratio mass spectrometer. This process is quantitative and does not generate isotopic fractionation. The sensitivity of this instrument allows the determination of isotope ratios of around 400 ng of a compound injected onto the column. Thus, the technique makes it possible to use a smaller sample compared with an elementary analyzer, where tens of micrograms are necessary. However, compared with a GC/C/IRMS, the sensitivity is not enhanced. Indeed, with this new interface, quantities of a few nanograms can be analyzed. At present, the IRM-LC/MS coupling does not make it possible to replace the GC/C/IRMS, in particular with regard to the analysis of trace compounds of, say, steroid hormones.

However, the IRM-LC/MS coupling does appear to represent a new technique of analysis for certain applications, such as the analysis of organic acids in plants[18], or underivatized amino acids,[15] or the analysis of RNA.[19] The advantage of this new technique remains in the analysis of complex molecules such as conjugate compounds (e.g. sulfates or glucuronides), but it also gives ability to analyze the majority of molecules without going through the derivation step (as

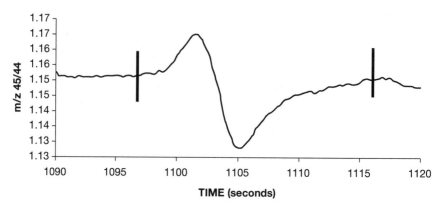

Figure 6.8 A typical IRMS chromatogram trace for *m/z* 45/44.

is needed in GC/C/IRMS). However, the sensitivity of this interface remains a weak point for the analysis of steroids at trace levels. Even if certain stages in the extraction and purification method usually used in GC/C/IRMS can be dispensed with in analysis via IRM-LC/MS (hydrolyses, derivation), the quantities of analytes of 250 ng for biological matrices seem difficult to reach.

15 Detection of testosterone doping by IRMS

In 1990, Southan *et al.*[20] published a study indicating that synthetic, pharmaceutical testosterone seemed to have a $^{13}C/^{12}C$ isotope ratio different from that of endogenous compounds biosynthesized by the human body. This observation was based on the fact that endogenous steroid hormones and those synthesized industrially do not have the same origins.

The hemisynthesis of steroids is the method most used by the pharmaceutical industry. The plants used as a raw material for these syntheses are, for example, phytosterols from soy plants[21] (Figure 6.9a). Diosgenine, a Mexican plant of the Dioscorea family which contains a glucoside steroid in its tubers, can also be used. These plants all have a C_3 photosynthetic cycle. They will thus have a naturally lower ^{13}C content. Therefore, the pharmaceutical compounds synthesized from these plants as starting material will be naturally depleted in ^{13}C. The endogenous hormones are biosynthesized from cholesterol in the body, itself biosynthesized from ingested food. These molecules also have a vegetable origin, but starting from precursors drawn from food. The isotope composition of the endogenous steroids is thus a reflection of the ^{13}C content of the many plants composing our food and that of the animals constituting our protein intake. Consequently, these endogenous molecules whose isotope composition comes from a mixture of various vegetable origins, C_3 and/or C_4, will be enriched in ^{13}C compared to molecules coming from a vegetable source solely comprising C_3 plants. Conversely, exogenous steroids reflecting only one single source of carbon (C_3 plants) will be naturally depleted in ^{13}C compared to the endogenous

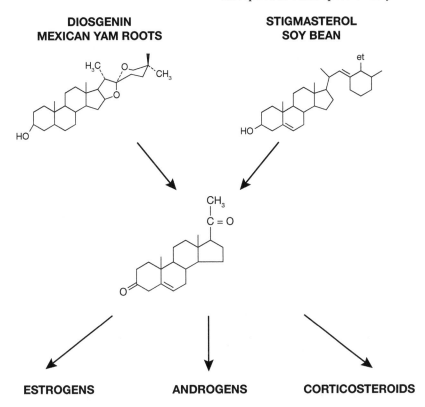

Figure 6.9a The main raw materials from C_3 plants used to hemisynthesize steroids.

molecules coming from a mixture of C_3 and/or C_4 plants. It is this difference in abundance in ^{13}C that will be highlighted by the isotopic analysis of carbon via GC/C/IRMS to identify the origin of the steroid hormones.

These two routes are illustrated in Figure 6.9b. To summarize, the proportion of ^{13}C in the endogenous molecule depends on the animal's food, while that of the exogenous molecule depends on the plant used at the time of organic synthesis of the active ingredient. Thus, in the case of an athlete who uses testosterone, the ^{13}C/^{12}C ratio of metabolites will be the result of a mixture of these two sources (endogenous and exogenous). It is by comparing the proportion of ^{13}C contained in the metabolites with that of an endogenous reference compound (ERC) – or, even better, with that of an endogenous precursor – that one will be able to determine whether a substance was or was not administered. If the difference in the isotope composition of the "precursor metabolites" is not significantly different, the analyst will be able to rule out the administration of an exogenous substance – or at least, to say that the evidence is insufficient. When the difference becomes significant, the assumption that a steroid is being administered becomes increasingly tenable.

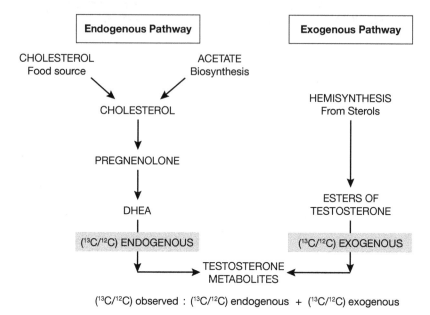

Figure 6.9b The two different pathways for arriving at testosterone, its precursors and its metabolites.

16 Application to the control of doping in the sporting field

16.1 *Study of testosterone (metabolites and precursors)*

The first studies on the origin of testosterone by GC/C/IRMS date from the beginning of the 1990s.[20] These studies related primarily to the measurement of exogenous testosterone in humans. Beginning in 1990, Southan *et al.* showed for the first time that the $^{13}C/^{12}C$ ratio was significantly different for endogenous and exogenous testosterone respectively. Thereafter, Becchi *et al.*[22] proposed the first method by which to differentiate exogenous and endogenous testosterone in the sporting field. The method involved comparison of differences in the $^{13}C/^{12}C$ ratio of androstanediols (metabolites of testosterone and cholesterol) in the urine; consequently, the detection of testosterone administration becomes possible.

This technique represents a complement to the anti-doping control method usually used for testosterone, which is based on measuring the concentrations of testosterone (T) and epitestosterone (E) in the urine by GC/MS. A T/E ratio is thus calculated, which should not exceed 6 in the case of a negative result or a negative control. Aguilera *et al.* proposed in 1996 a complementary study of how the administration of testosterone would affect the $^{13}C/^{12}C$ ratios of its metabolites in urine.[23,24] The measurement of the isotope ratio difference of two precursors (cholesterol and 5-androstene-3β,17α-diol and of two metabolites (5α- and 5β-androstane-3β,17α-diol) additional to testosterone made it possible to make a statistical study and thereby to differentiate the control samples from those who had had testosterone administered to them. The method suggested gives results comparable with those obtained with the measurement of T/E ratio. According to the authors, it could be used as a confirmatory method to avoid false positives and false negatives given by T/E ratio measurements. This observation was confirmed by Horning *et al.* in 1996, who presented this new approach at an annual congress on anti-doping control in athletes.[25] The study undertaken by the author compares the results obtained by the traditional method (T/E ratio) with those obtained via GC/C/IRMS measurement after testosterone administration. The study showed that the T/E ratio increases rapidly after the administration (from 1.1 to 22.2 in 2 hours), then decreases to values lower than 6 after 6 hours. The $\delta^{13}C/^{12}C$ values of testosterone were also rapidly affected (from –24.4 to –28.1‰ in 2 hours), but the return to the normal values took longer. The same result was observed by Aguilera *et al.* (2000), who developed and validated a faster method requiring only 2 mL of urine to measure the $^{13}C/^{12}C$ ratio of the androsterone and etiocholanolone.[26] Moreover, to solve ambiguities in the interpretation of the results obtained by measurement of T/E ratio, Aguilera *et al.* (2001) analyzed different T/E ratios greater than 6. By measuring the $^{13}C/^{12}C$ of metabolites and precursors of testosterone, the study showed that in certain cases even if T/E is greater than 6, that does not necessarily mean that exogenous testosterone has been administered.[27] Furthermore, a T/E ratio lower than 6 can sometimes be obtained if the subject has taken synthetic epitestosterone. To avoid this problem, Aguilera *et al.* (2002) proposed a method for the detection of epitestosterone by GC/C/IRMS. These authors showed that the abuse of steroids could be detected in athletes having a T/E ratio of 1.1.[28]

16.2 Extension of the method to measurements of other steroid hormones

Subsequently, the use of GC/C/IRMS in the world of anti-doping control in sports widened to include all of the natural steroid hormones. In 1997, Shackleton *et al.* presented a method that measured the $^{13}C/^{12}C$ ratio of androstanediols and 5-androstenediols in order to highlight any exogenous administration of dihydrotestosterone (DHT), epitestosterone or dehydroepiandrosterone (DHEA).[29] This measurement of $\delta^{13}C/^{12}C$ values also makes it possible to interpret the effects of steroid hormones on metabolism. Shackleton *et al.* emphasize the influence of the administration of steroid hormones based on the detection of several androstanediols and androstanediols present in urine. These results allowed the targeting of specific molecules to be analyzed when various different exogenous substances have been used. In addition to this, Horning *et al.* (1997) presented a metabolic study of DHT and testosterone using GC/C/IRMS.[30] After administration of DHT, various

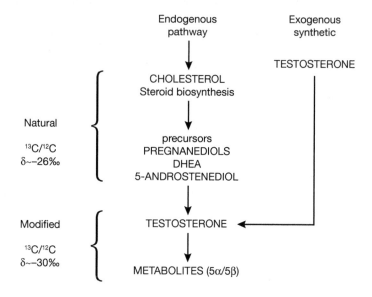

Figure 6.10 Endogenous and exogenous origin of testosterone and its metabolites, and the influence of an exogenous administration of testosterone on the $^{13}C/^{12}C$ ratios of the metabolites.

metabolites of testosterone were affected in different ways. Androsterone (5α) and the 5α-androstane-3α,17β-diol were depleted in ^{13}C after injection, whereas etiocholanolone (5β) and 5β-androstane-3α,17β-diol were not affected. This study showed that it was important to measure the $\delta^{13}C/^{12}C$ values for several metabolites, because, depending on metabolism, not all metabolites will be affected in the same way. With this point in mind Shackleton *et al.* (1997) measured the $\delta^{13}C/^{12}C$ values of androstanediols (5α- and 5β-androstane-3α,17β-diols) after administration of testosterone enanthate.[31] Androstanediols show a significant variation in $\delta^{13}C/^{12}C$ values after treatment, while precursors do not show significant variation. Moreover, Shackleton *et al.* (1997)[29] and Aguilera *et al.* (1999)[24] proposed the possibility of using 5β-pregnane-3α, 20α-diol as an endogenous reference compound for the detection of testosterone administration.

16.3 Study of DHEA and its metabolites and precursors

DHEA is also one of the unauthorized steroid hormones listed by the medical commission of the Olympic International Committee (IOC) and the World Anti-Doping Agency (WADA). However, this substance is widely diffused in the United States, where it can be bought over the counter. This is why $\delta^{13}C/^{12}C$ values were also used to detect DHEA abuse. Horning *et al.* (1997)[30] and Shackleton *et al.* (1997)[31] studied the influence of the administration of DHEA on various androstanediols and androstenediols. They concluded that one of the major metabolites of DHEA is the 5-androstene-3β, 17β-diol, which was a relevant marker, along with other androstanediols. If the $\delta^{13}C/^{12}C$ values for metabolites were depleted in ^{13}C, that means that DHEA was used. If only the androstanediols are depleted in ^{13}C, a suspicion of administration of another androgen has to be considered.

Ueki *et al.* (1999)[32] carried out a study of ten suspect urine samples from athletes who had taken part in the Seventeenth Winter Olympics in Nagano. These authors showed that the concentration of steroid hormones (in DHEA more particularly) is not directly related to an exogenous input. Indeed, certain athletes had strong concentrations of DHEA, whereas the isotope ratio values of this substance were not particularly impoverished and not appreciably different from those of the endogenous compound of reference (pregnanediol). To confirm the administration of DHEA, Saudan *et al.* (2004)[33] proposed to follow the $^{13}C/^{12}C$ ratio of the 16(5α)-androsten-3α-ol, a metabolite of pregnenolone but independent of DHEA. By comparison of the isotope ratio from these two analytes, the authors emphasize the interest in regarding 16(5α)-androsten-3α-ol as an endogenous compound of reference for the detection of administration of DHEA and/or testosterone. These same authors confirmed this result in 2005 with an article showing the influence of the administration of pregnenolone on the metabolites and precursors of testosterone.[34] This study revealed a modification of the isotopic $^{13}C/^{12}C$ ratios of principal metabolites of testosterone as well as 16(5α)-androsten-3α-ol. An important remark in this study is that the administration of pregnenolone does not affect measurements of the T/E ratio that are carried out for the purpose of detecting doping. Once more, GC/C/IRMS brought additional information and often saving cases within the framework of anti-doping control. It was by the study of the evolution of the isotopic ratio of various molecules observed via GC/MS that Cawley *et al.* (2004)[35] showed that there were steroids likely to be regarded as markers of an administration of DHEA. Indeed, these authors were interested in 3α, 5-cyclo-5α-androstan-6β-ol-17-one, whose concentrations increase considerably after the taking of DHEA. They were able to show a significant impoverishment of this molecule after treatment. Cawley *et al.* (2005) carried out another study of the metabolism of DHEA by measuring the isotope ratios of a precursor (11-keto-etiocholanolone) and two metabolites (etiocholanolone (compound in 5β) and androsterone (compound in 5α)) after administration of DHEA. By comparison of the isotopic ratios differences between $\delta^{13}C$ etiocholanolone and $\delta^{13}C$ androsterone, the author emphasizes this finding as a specific mark of an exogenous administration of DHEA.[36] Indeed, etiocholanolone remains depleted in ^{13}C for longer than androsterone after administration of DHEA, whereas this phenomenon was not observed in the studies where androstenedione (Δ^4) and testosterone had been used.

16.4 Study of corticosteroids

In parallel with methods developed for androgens, many methods were proposed for the analysis of a variety of hormones by GC/C/IRMS. The corticosteroids, whose use is regulated by WADA, were studied by Becchi *et al.*[37] The $\delta^{13}C/^{12}C$ values of endogenous metabolites such as tetrahydrocortisone (THE) and tetrahydrocortisol (THF) were compared with those of synthetic preparations of cortisol and cortisone. The results obtained were similar to the observations made for androgens: the exogenous molecules have $\delta^{13}C/^{12}C$ values significantly different from those of the endogenous molecules. However, a nuance in the results was observed for cortisone. Depending on the supplier, the isotopic measurements taken revealed either an enrichment in ^{13}C ($\delta^{13}C = -14‰$) or an impoverishment in ^{13}C ($\delta^{13}C = -26‰$). These observations were explained by the different origins of the raw materials used for the synthesis of these molecules. However, in both cases these results remain significantly different from the $\delta^{13}C/^{12}C$ values of the endogenous compounds ($\delta^{13}C = -22‰$ on average). A similar study was carried out by Bourgogne *et al.*[38] The same results were obtained for synthetic molecules: either significantly impoverished ($\delta^{13}C$ sometimes as low as $-33‰$) or significantly enriched (up to $-17‰$) compared with the endogenous molecules ($-23‰$ on average). The complementary analysis by GC/C/IRMS of metabolites of THE and THF (after oxidation) of a subject who had been treated with hydrocortisone made it possible to confirm the effectiveness of the method for the corticosteroids (an average of $-28‰$ was found for these metabolites).

16.5 Study of 19-norsteroids

Other molecules such as 19-norsteroids were studied by GC/C/IRMS in order to determine the exogenous or, alternatively, endogenous origins of one of the principal metabolites of nandrolone, 19-norandrosterone[39,40] However, the urinary concentrations observed for this molecule were often too low; no direct analysis of samples could be carried out. Only substances of reference of the 19-norsteroid type could be measured. Desroches *et al.*[41] have proposed a purification method, namely immunoaffinity chromatography, for the study of these compounds. They claim that this technique is promising for the analysis of 19-norandrosterone.

16.6 Application to horse racing

Concerning tests for equine doping, very few isotopic studies based on the $^{13}C/^{12}C$ ratio of steroid hormones have been carried out. Some preliminary results have been published by Aguilera *et al.*[42] concerning a study aimed at determining the origin of cortisol in horses using GC/C/IRMS.

16.7 Application to the control of the illicit use of hormones in farm animals

Similar studies were carried out with animals in order to underline the illegal use of steroid hormones in animal breeding. In 1998, Mason *et al.*[43] published the results of a study in which they measured the $^{13}C/^{12}C$ isotopic ratio of 5β-androstane-3α,17α-diol (the principal testosterone metabolite found in bovine bile) and compared it with the isotopic ratio of cholesterol (an endogenous molecule) after treatment of an animal with testosterone esters. They found a significant difference in the $\delta^{13}C/^{12}C$ values for cholesterol compared to androstane between treated and nontreated animals. Ferchaud *et al.* (1998)[44] developed a method that allowed the control of testosterone abuse in farm animals. Indeed, by comparison of the isotope ratios of the metabolites of testosterone to those found in a precursor such as DHEA, the administration of exogenous testosterone can be proved. More recently, in 2000, Ferchaud and coworkers published work showing the influence of food and the age of the animal on the $^{13}C/^{12}C$ isotopic ratios of steroid hormones.[45,46] Depending on what the animal is fed, the isotopic ratios of the metabolites and precursors of testosterone will be enriched (maize) or will be impoverished (hay). However, even within the framework of a foodstuff of the hay variety where the isotopic ratios will be reduced the detection of exogenous testosterone use remains achievable. Ferchaud also emphasized the influence of age on the metabolite–precursor isotopic ratios after testosterone administration.[45–47] Thus, the adult animal seems to show less marked isotope ratios between metabolites and precursors than does an 8-month-old heifer. In 2005, Balizs *et al.* studied the influence of animal food on the $^{13}C/^{12}C$ isotopic ratios of hormones in bovine urine.[48] The results show that in extreme cases, for example in the case of animals fed exclusively with type C_3 plants or type plants C_4, the isotopic deviations of the metabolites can vary from –19‰ to –32‰. Thus, within the framework of a food based exclusively on type C_3 plants, with the isotopic deviation of the metabolites ranging from –24‰ to –32‰, verification of exogenous testosterone administration becomes delicate. Additional and extended studies in this field have been carried out by others.[49–51]

17 Conclusion

After more than a decade of basic research and investigations into applications of steroid analysis, IRMS has become one of the most powerful tools for detecting doping in sport. This technique, coupled with gas chromatography and combustion (GC/C/IRMS), measures the carbon isotope ratio in a steroid, relative to an international convention reference standard. The ratio of $^{13}C/^{12}C$ can be measured with high accuracy and precision by an isotope ratio mass spectrometer. Consequently, very small differences in the abundance of ^{13}C can be detected, allowing the differentiation of various sources of carbon arising from natural and/or pharmaceutical steroids. New applications are under development, as well as new technologies to improve steroid detection. Nonetheless, the implementation of this technique at the trace level remains a challenge. The study of steroid metabolism using GC/C/IRMS has not been considered in the appropriate fashion either, which also includes extending the approach to the mass balance required for drug analysis by the pharmaceutical industry, because of the delay in the development of LC/C/IRMS.

Acknowledgements

I dedicate this chapter to my mentor Dr Michel Becchi. With thanks to Dr Thomas E Chapman for all his help with reviewing this chapter and Dr Corinne Buisson for her contribution.

18 References

1 Platzner IT, Habfast K, Walder AJ, Goetz A. In: Wineforder JD, ed. *Modern isotope ratio mass spectrometry*. New York: J. Wiley; 1997.

2 Coplen TB. Reporting of stable hydrogen, carbon, and oxygen isotopic abundances. *Pure and Applied Chemistry*. 1984; 66: 273–6.

3 Coplen TB. New guidelines for reporting stable hydrogen, carbon, and oxygen isotope-ratio data. *Geochimica et Cosmochimica Acta*. 1996; 60(17): 3359–60.

4 Skoog DA, West DM, Holler FJ. *Chimie analytique*. 7th ed. Paris: De Boeck Université.

5 Meier-Augenstein W. The chromatographic side of isotope ratio mass spectrometry: pitfalls and answers. *LC-GC International*. 1997; 17–25.

6 Meier-Augenstein W. Applied gas chromatography coupled to isotope ratio mass spectrometry. *Journal of Chromatography A*. 1999; 842: 351–71.

7 Craig H. Isotopic standards for carbon and oxygen and correction factors for mass-spectrometric analysis of carbon dioxide. *Geochimica et Cosmochimica Acta*. 1957; 12: 133–49.

8 Eakin P, Fallick A, Gerc J. Some instrumental effects in the determination of stable carbon isotope ratios by gas chromatography-isotope ratio mass spectrometry. *Chemical Geology*. 1992; 101: 71–9.

9 Costes C, Bourdu R, Champigny ML, Jolivet E, Moyse A, Bonnemain JL, Chartier P, Monties B, Aussenac G, Giraud G, de Cormis L., *Photosynthèse et production végétale*. Paris: Bordas.

10 Aguilera R. Differenciation entre testostérone endogène et testostérone exogène par analyse isotopique du carbone: application au contrôle antidopage. Doctoral thesis, Université de Lyon, Service Central d'Analyse CNRS, 1996.

11 Buisson C. Développement d'une stratégie analytique basée sur la spectrométrie de masse de rapport isotopique appliquée au contrôle de l'usage frauduleux d'hormones stéroïdes en élevage. Doctoral thesis, Université de Nantes, 2005.

12 Shahidi NT. A review of chemistry, biological action, and clinical applications of anabolic-androgenic steroids. *Clinical Therapeutics*. 2001; 23(9): 1355–90.

13 Meier-Augenstein W, Watt P, Langhans C. Influence of gas chromatographic parameters on measurement of $^{13}C/^{12}C$ isotope ratios by gas–liquid chromatography–

combustion isotope ratio mass spectrometry. I. *Journal of Chromatography A*. 1996; 752: 233–41.

14 Santrock & Hayes. Isotopic Compositor Analyser. Patent 5314827, vol. 11 (11): 583. European Patent Application.

15 Juchelka D, Krummen M. IRM-LC/MS: $\delta^{13}C$ analysis of underivatized amino acids. Application note 30065; Thermo Electron Corporation, 2005.

16 Osborn BL, Abramson FP. *Proceedings of the Forty-third ASMS Conference Mass Spectrometry and Allied Topics, Atlanta*, 1994; 875.

17 Caimi RJ, Brenna JT. 1997. Quantitative evaluation of carbon isotopic fractionation during reversed-phase high-performance liquid chromatography. *Journal of Chromatography A*. 1997; 757: 307–10.

18 Hettmann E and Gleixner G. IRM-LC/MS: $\delta^{13}C$ analysis of organic acids in plants. Application note 30075, Thermo Electron Corporation, 2005.

19 MacGregor B, Friedman A. IRM-LC/MS: $\delta^{13}C$ analysis of RNA. Application note 30055; Thermo Electron Corporation, 2005.

20 Southan G, Mallat A, Jumeau J, Craig S, Poojara N, Mitchell D. Programme and Abstracts of the Second International Symposium on Applied Mass Spectrometry in the Health Sciences, Barcelona, 1990 April 16–19: 306.

21 Gaignault J-C, Bidet D, Gaillard M, Perronnet J. *Stérols et stéroïdes*. Paris: Ellipses, 1997; 155–9.

22 Becchi M, Aguilera R, Farizon Y, Flament MM, Casabianca H, James P. Gas chromatography/combustion/isotope-ratio mass spectrometry analysis of urinary steroids to detect misuse of testosterone in sport. *Rapid Communications in Mass Spectrometry*. 1994; 8: 304–8.

23 Aguilera R, Becchi M, Casabianca H. Improved method of detection of testosterone abuse by gas chromatography/combustion/isotope ratio mass spectrometry analysis of urinary steroids. *Journal of Mass Spectrometry* 31: 1996; 169–76.

24 Aguilera R, Catlin DH, Becchi M, Phillips A, Wang C. Screening urine for exogenous testosterone by isotope ratio mass spectrometric analysis of one prenianediol and two androstanediols. *Journal of Chromatography B: Analytical Techniques in the Biomedical and Life Services*. 1999; 727: 95–105.

25 Horning S, Machnik M, Schanzer W, Hilkert A, Oesselmann J. Detection of exogenous testosterone by $^{13}C/^{12}C$ analysis. *Recent advances in doping analysis (4), Proceedings of the Fourteenth Cologne Workshop on Dope Analysis*. Cologne: Sport und Buch Strauß, 1996; 275–83.

26 Aguilera R, Chapman TE, Catlin DH. Rapid screening assay for measuring urinary androsterone and etiocholanolone $\delta^{13}C$(‰) values by gas chromatography/combustion/isotope ratio mass spectrometry. *Rapid Communications in Mass Spectrometry*. 2000; 14: 2294–9.

27 Aguilera R, Chapman TE, Starcevic B, Hatton CK, Catlin DH. Performance characteristics of a carbon isotope ratio method for detecting doping with testosterone based on urine diols: controls and athletes with elevated testosterone/epitestosterone ratios. *Clinical Chemistry*. 2001; 47(2): 292–300.

28 Aguilera R, Hatton CK, Catlin DH. Detection of epitestosterone doping by isotope ratio mass spectrometry. *Clinical Chemistry* 48(4): 629–36.

29 Shackleton CHL, Phillips A, Chang T, Li Y. Confirming testosterone administration by isotope ratio mass spectrometric analysis of urinary androstanediols. *Steroids*. 1997; 62 : 379–87.

30 Horning S, Geyer H, Flenker U, Schanzer W. Detection of exogenous steroids by

$^{13}C/^{12}C$ analysis. *Recent advances in doping analysis (5), Proceeding of the Fifteenth Cologne Workshop on Dope Analysis.* Cologne: Sport und Buch Strauβ, 1997: 135–48.

31 Shackleton CHL, Roitman E, Phillips A, Chang T. Androstanediol and 5-androstendiol profiling for detecting exogenously administred dihydrotestosterone, epitestosterone, and dehydroepiandrosterone: potential use in gas chromatography isotope ratio mass spectrometry. *Steroids.* 1997; 62: 665–73.

32 Ueki M, Okano M. Analysis of exogenous dehydroepiandrosterone excretion in urine by gas chromatography/combustion/isotope ratio mass spectrometry. *Rapid Communications in Mass Spectrometry.* 1999; 13: 2237–43.

33 Saudan C, Baume N, Mangin P, Saugy M. Urinary analysis of 16(5α)-androsten-3α-ol by gas chromatography/combustion/isotope ratio mass spectrometry: implications in anti-doping analysis. *Journal of Chromatography B: Analytical Techniques in the Biomedical and Life Sciences.* 2004; 810: 157–64.

34 Saudan CDA, Sottas PE, Mangin P, Saugy A. Urinary markers of oral pregnenolone administration. *Steroids.* 2005; 70: 179–83.

35 Cawley AT, Hine ER, Trout GJ, George AV, Kazlauskas R. Searching for new markers of endogenous steroid administration in athletes: "looking outside the metabolic box." *Forensic Science International.* 2004; 143: 103–14.

36 Cawley AT, Kazlauskas R, Trout GJ, Rogerson JH, George AV. Isotopic fraction-ation of endogenous anabolic androgenic steroids and its relationship to doping control in sports. *Journal of Chromatographic Science.* 2005; 43: 32–8.

37 Becchi M, Perret F, Forest D, Mathurin JC, De Ceaurriz J. Carbone isotope ratio mass spectrometry of endogenous corticosteroids. *Proceedings of the Seventeenth Cologne Workshop on Dope Analysis.* Cologne: Sport und Buch Strauβ, 1999; 233–40.

38 Bourgogne EHV, Mathurin JC, Becchi M, De Ceaurriz J. Detection of exogenous intake of natural corticosteroids by GC/C/IRMS: application to misuse in sport. *Rapid Communications in Mass Spectrometry.* 2000; 14: 2343–7.

39 Mathurin JC, Herrou V, Bourgogne E, Pascaud L, De Ceaurriz J. Gas chromatography-combustion-isotope ratio mass spectrometry analysis of 19-norsteroids: application to the detection of a nandrolone metabolite in urine. *Journal of Chromatography B: Analytical Techniques in the Biomedical and Life Sciences.* 2001; 759: 267–75.

40 Mathurin JC, Bourgogne E, Barrault Y, De Ceaurriz J. Différenciation de l'origine exogène ou endogène de produits dopants par l'analyse isotopique du carbone. *Revue Française des Laboratoires.* 2001; 331: 29–36.

41 Desroches MC, M.J., Richard Y, Delahaut P, De Ceaurriz J. Urinary 19-norandrosterone purification by immunoaffinity chromatography: application to GC/C/IRMS analysis. *Rapid Communications in Mass Spectrometry.* 2002; 16: 370–4.

42 Aguilera R, Becchi M, Mateus L, Popot, M.A, Bonnaire Y, Casabianca H, Hatton CK. Detection of exogenous hydrocortisone in horse urine by gas chromatography-combustion-carbon isotope ratio mass spectrometry. *Journal of Chromatography B: Analytical Techniques in the Biomedical and Life Sciences.* 1997; 702: 85.

43 Mason PM, Hall SE, Gilmour I, Houghton E, Pillinger C, Seymour MA. The use of stable carbon isotope analysis to detect the abuse of testosterone in cattle. *Analyst.* 1998; 123: 2405–8.

44 Ferchaud V, Le Bizec B, Monteau F, André F. Determination of the exogenous

character of testosterone in bovine urine by gas chromatography-combustion-isotope-ratio-mass spectrometry. *Analyst*. 1998; 123: 2617–20.

45 Ferchaud V, Le Bizec B, Monteau F, André F. Characterization of exogenous tesosterone in livestock by gas chromatography/combustion/isotope ratio mass spectrometry: influence of feeding and age. *Rapid Communications in Mass Spectrometry*. 2000; 14: 652–6.

46 Ferchaud V, Le Bizec B, Monteau F, André F. Natural steroid hormones: GC/C/IRMS: the unequivocal solution to demonstrate their illegal use? *EuroResidue IV*; 2000 May 8–10, Velhoven, the Netherlands.

47 Ferchaud V. Détermination par GC/C/IRMS du caractère exogène des hormones stéroïdes naturelles: application au dépistage de l'usage frauduleux de la testostérone et de ses esters en élevage. Doctoral thesis, Université de Nantes, Faculté des sciences et techniques.

48 Balizs G, Jainz A, Horvatovich P. Investigation of the feeding effect on the $^{13}C/^{12}C$ isotope ratio of the hormones in bovine urine using gas chromatography/combustion isotope ratio mass spectrometry. *Journal of Chromatography A*. 2005; 1067: 323–30.

49 Buisson C, Hebestreit M, Preiss Weigert A, Heinrich K, Fry H, Flenker U, Banneke S, Prevost S, André F, Schänzer W, Houghton E, Le Bizec B. Application of stable carbon istope analysis to detection of 17β-estradiol administration to cattle. *Journal of Chromatography A*. 2005; 1093: 69–80.

50 Hebestreit M, Flenker U, Buisson C, André F, Le Bizec B, Fry H, Lang M, Preiss Weigert A, Heinrich K, Hird S, Schänzer W. Application of stable carbon isotope analysis to the detection of testosterone administration to cattle. *Journal of Agricultural and Food Chemistry*. 2006; 54: 2850–8.

51 Prévost S, Nicol T, Monteau F, André F, Le Bizec B. GC/C/IRMS to control the misuse of androgens in breeding animals: new derivatisation method applied to testosterone metabolites and precursors in urine samples. *Rapid Communications in Mass Spectrometry*. 2001; 15: 2509–14.

Additional recommended literature not included in the text

Aguilera, R, Becchi M, Grenot C, Casabianca H, Hatton CK. Detection of testosterone misuse: comparison of two chromatographic sample preparation methods for gas chromatographic–combustion/isotope ratio mass spectrometric analysis. *Journal of Chromatography B: Analytical Techniques in the Biomedical and Life Sciences*. 1996; 687: 43–53.

de la Torre X. $^{13}C/^{12}C$ isotope ratio MS analysis of testosterone, in chemicals and pharmaceutical preparations. *Pharmaceutical and Biomedical Analysis*. 2001; 24: 645–50.

IUPAC Commission on Atomic Weights and Isotopic Abundances. Atomic weights of the elements 1993. *Pure and Applied Chemistry* 1994; 66: 2423–44.

Jasper JP, Westenberger BJ, Spencer JA, Buhse LF, Nasr M, Stable isotope characterization of active pharmaceutical ingredients. *Journal of Pharmaceutical and Biomedical Analysis*. 2004; 35: 21–30.

Ueki, M, Okano, M. Doping with naturally occurring steroids. *Toxicology*. 1999; 18(2): 177–95.

7 Stimulants, diuretics and masking of doping in sport

Richard L Hilderbrand

1 Introduction

The desire to win has existed in athletes since time immemorial. This desire has fueled the use of substances to enhance performance irrespective of the ability of a substance to actually improve performance. Reports of use of various herbal materials, even in ancient times, exist and indicate that stimulants have been a preferred category of substances for performance enhancement. In recent years, the remarkable developments in the pharmaceutical industry have only fueled the use of performance-enhancing substances, and the use of medications and methods to enhance performance has become widespread among athletes and the general population. During the 1930s, amphetamines came into favor as a stimulant, and allegedly were used in various sports through the 1940s and 1950s. In the 1952 Olympic Winter Games, several speed skaters became ill and needed medical attention after taking amphetamines.[1] The event that caught the attention of the International Olympic Committee and sports enthusiasts worldwide was the televised death in the 1967 Tour de France of the British cyclist Tom Simpson as recorded in *Put me back on my bike*.[2] Following several years of development of anti-doping programs, an independent organization, the World Anti-Doping Agency (WADA), was established to implement and harmonize anti-doping efforts worldwide.

2 The World Anti-Doping Program

The World Anti-Doping Program consists of the World Anti-Doping Code (the Code),[3] which establishes policy, and several international standards. The two international standards that are salient to this chapter are the International Standard for Therapeutic Use Exemptions[4] and the Prohibited List International Standard.[5] These standards are written to harmonize the therapeutic use exemption request process and the substances prohibited across all International Federations and other relevant anti-doping organizations throughout the world.

The International Standard for Therapeutic Use Exemptions (TUEs) allows an athlete who has a legitimate medical need for the use of an otherwise prohibited substance or method to submit a request to use that particular treatment. The International Standard for TUEs includes the criteria for allowing the exemption, the application process, and a procedure for appeals to decisions. There are two types of TUEs. The first is an Abbreviated TUE, which is a notification of use only. If it is filled out properly and completely, it is effective upon receipt at the relevant anti-doping organization. The Abbreviated TUE may be used only for corticosteroids administered by inhalation or local injection and certain β_2-agonists that are permitted by inhalation for respiratory conditions. The Abbreviated TUE relies on the signature of the physician, and only in certain cases does it require documentation by medical records. The second type of TUE is the Standard TUE, which applies to all other prohibited substances and methods and must be supported by complete medical documentation. The Standard TUE must be submitted and approved prior to the use of the prohibited medication or method where the rules of sport are enforced. In the case of an emergency that requires the use of a prohibited medication or method to protect the health of the athlete, an Emergency TUE must be submitted on the Standard TUE form and an attachment containing the full medical documentation of the situation requiring the emergency treatment and of the medical treatment provided. The decision on the approval or denial of an Emergency TUE is generally made after the fact of the use of the prohibited medication.

The Prohibited List International Standard (the List) is updated annually to be effective the first day of each year and otherwise as required, and must be monitored to ensure all stakeholders have the most recent information. The List includes the categories of substances and methods that are prohibited and specifies whether the substance or method is prohibited at all times or only in-competition. The List is compiled by a committee convened by WADA and the proposed list is then circulated for comment. The List is not exhaustive in that several categories of substances are "open" and may include "other substances with a similar chemical structure or similar biological effect(s)" that are not specifically named. The inclusion of a substance or method on the List is not subject to appeal by the athlete in the case of a doping violation. This chapter covers stimulants, β_2-agonists, diuretics, and their relationship to sport – including the procedures to file an abbreviated TUE or request a Standard TUE.

Text in this chapter from the WADA Prohibited List was taken directly from the List. No changes or corrections have been made by the author.

3 Stimulants (prohibited list – category S6)

All stimulants (including both their (D- & L-) optical isomers where relevant) are prohibited, except imidazole derivatives for topical use and those stimulants included in the 2008 Monitoring Program*.

Stimulants include:

Adrafinil, adrenaline**, amfepramone, amiphenazole, amphetamine, amphetaminil, benzphetamine, benzylpiperazine, bromantan, cathine***, clobenzorex, cocaine, cropropamide, crotetamide, cyclazodone, dimethylamphetamine, ephedrine****, etamivan, etilamphetamine, etilefrine, famprofazone, fenbutrazate, fencamfamin, fencamine, fenetylline, fenfluramine, fenproporex, furfenorex, heptaminol, isometheptene, levmethamfetamine, meclofenoxate, mefenorex, mephentermine, mesocarb, methamphetamine (D-), methylenedioxyamphetamine, methylenedioxymethamphetamine, *p*-methylamphetamine, methylephedrine****, methylphenidate, modafinil, nikethamide, norfenefrine, norfenfluramine, octopamine, ortetamine, oxilofrine, parahydroxyamphetamine, pemoline, pentetrazol, phendimetrazine, phenmetrazine, phenpromethamine, phentermine, 4-phenylpiracetam (carphedon), prolintane, propylhexedrine, selegiline, sibutramine, strychnine, tuaminoheptane and other substances with a similar chemical structure or similar biological effect(s).

* The following substances included in the 2008 Monitoring Program (bupropion, caffeine, phenylephrine, phenylpropanolamine, pipradol, pseudoephedrine, synephrine) are not considered as *Prohibited Substances*.

** Adrenaline associated with local anaesthetic agents or by local administration (e.g. nasal, ophthalmologic) is not prohibited.

*** Cathine is prohibited when its concentration in urine is greater than 5 micrograms per milliliter.

**** Each of ephedrine and methylephedrine is prohibited when its concentration in urine is greater than 10 micrograms per milliliter.

3.1 Status of stimulants in sport

During 2005, WADA received 509 reports of adverse findings for the use of stimulants (Table 7.1).[6] Of these findings, some may be multiple specimens for certain athletes due to multiple test sessions and some may be from athletes with an approved TUE (e.g. for ADD and ADHD). Therefore, the number of adverse analytical findings does not represent the number of athletes sanctioned for the use of a stimulant. The stimulants prohibited[5] by the WADA cover several types of substances and uses, including those such as amphetamine (which is listed as a Schedule II drug by the US Department of Justice, Drug Enforcement Agency, Controlled Substances Act),[7] prescription medications, over-the-counter medications and herbal substances (e.g. ephedrine).

Adrenaline (epinephrine) occurs naturally in the human body and is responsible for a wide range of effects related to the "fight or flight" response. Adrenaline acts through the stimulation of both α- and β-adrenoceptors, but does not cross the blood-brain barrier readily. The sympathomimetics such as amphetamine and 3,4-methylenedioxy-*N*-methylamphetamine (MDMA; Ecstasy) mimic the

Table 7.1 WADA adverse analytical findings for stimulants, 2005

Stimulant	Occurrence	Percentage within drug class
Amphetamine	194	38.1
Ephedrine	93	18.3
Cocaine metabolites	85	16.7
Methylphenidate	17	3.3
Cathine	14	2.8
Phentermine	14	2.8
MDMA	13	2.6
Methamphetamine	12	2.4
Heptaminol	11	2.2
MDA	8	1.6
Nikethamide	8	1.6
Benzylpiperazine	6	1.2
Carphedon	6	1.2
Etilefrine	4	0.8
Mephentermine	4	0.8
Norfenfluramine	3	0.6
Pemoline	3	0.6
Fenetylline	2	0.4
MDEA	2	0.4
Methylephedrine	2	0.4
Amfepramone	1	0.2
Clobenzorex	1	0.2
Etamivan	1	0.2
Methylamphetamine	1	0.2
Mesocarb	1	0.2
Modafinil	1	0.2
Parahydroxyamphetamine	1	0.2
Strychnine	1	0.2
TOTAL[a]	**509**	

a Some occurrences may be the result of multiple tests of the same athlete.

effects of epinephrine in the stimulation of the sympathetic nervous system. The indicators of stimulation due to release of epinephrine include anxiety, fear, restlessness, insomnia, confusion and irritability, and are largely a somatic response to the binding of adrenaline to receptors. Excessive stimulation of the sympathetic nervous system may produce side effects such as severe anxiety, dyspnea, hyperglycemia, restlessness, palpitations, tachycardia, tremors, sweating, hypersalivation, weakness, dizziness, headache and coldness of extremities – even at low doses.[8] The peripheral adverse effects of adrenaline are complex and mediated via its action on the various types of adrenergic receptors. Stimulation of α-adrenergic (mainly α_1) receptors produces vasoconstriction leading to hypertension, and this α-mediated hypertension may induce reflex bradycardia. On the other hand, stimulation of β_1-adrenergic receptors in the heart produces tachycardia and cardiac arrhythmias. Finally, stimulation of β_2 receptors produces vasodilatation with flushing and hypotension (more apparent if the vasoconstricting α-effects are blocked).[8]

Amphetamines and related compounds are notorious for producing health problems in athletes. Deaths from the cardiotoxicity of amphetamines are documented.[9] Although these drugs can produce both psychological and physical stimuli during athletic performance, it is important to note that the side effects can be harmful. The stimulants can be used to increase ability to train at a high level, to act as appetite suppressants to make weight, or to increase awareness and responsiveness. Medical uses include the treatment of narcolepsy, attention deficit disorder (ADD), attention deficit hyperactivity disorder (ADHD) and as an appetite suppressant.

Stimulants are only prohibited in-competition and may be used out-of-competition; however, their use must be discontinued prior to a competition to allow complete clearance from the body (including the urine). The stimulants listed above are prohibited by name; however, there is a phrase that includes substances with similar structure or function as being prohibited, which makes this an open class of substances. The use of a stimulant (including ADD medications) in-competition requires an approved Standard TUE. Some of the stimulants are subject to a concentration threshold that must be exceeded before the laboratory result is reported as an adverse finding.

3.2 *ADD/ADHD medications*

The most commonly prescribed medications to treat ADD and ADHD (e.g. Ritalin, Adderall and Concerta) are prohibited stimulants. These medications are prohibited and tested in-competition only and athletes prescribed these medications may, in consultation with their physician, discontinue use in advance of competition in order for the medication to clear their system (including the urine). If an athlete requires the use of a stimulant in-competition to treat ADD/ADHD, an exemption may be requested through the Therapeutic Use Exemption process. Prior to use in-competition, the request must be approved and the athlete notified of the approval.

For a TUE to be considered for the use of an ADD or ADHD medication, there are basic medical information requirements:

- A thorough clinical history, including the initial report(s) that led to the diagnosis of ADD/ADHD, discussion of the measures used and their interpretation, age of onset and family history of related diagnoses.
- The results of any laboratory testing that was done during the evaluation.
- A description of the deficit in physical or mental performance exhibited by the athlete and, if treatment is ongoing, how the proposed medication improved that performance.
- Observations of consequences when the medication is not taken for a period of time.
- Evidence that allowed medications have been considered or tried and that the outcome of use of the allowed medications is such that the prohibited medication must be used. (The treating physician must justify the need for the stimulant medication.)

- Any clinical, psychological, educational or consultative reports with comments on related performance issues such as anxiety or depression.
- A statement provided by the athlete outlining how he or she feels when the medication is being taken and not taken. This statement is helpful to the physicians, and should be written by the athlete, not written by parents over the athlete's signature.

Recently the FDA[10] directed the manufacturers of all drug products approved for the treatment of ADHD to provide information to patients on the possible cardiovascular risks and adverse psychiatric symptoms that may result from the use of the ADHD medications and to advise on what precautions may be taken. The manufacturers of the 15 medication brand names involved had previously been required to modify labeling of the products to warn of potential adverse cardiovascular or psychiatric events.

3.3 Metabolism of medications to amphetamines

Athletes should be aware that a number of medications listed as stimulants on the 2008 Prohibited List are metabolized by the body to produce amphetamine or methamphetamine. The laboratory will detect the original drug or the amphetamine(s) and the result will be an adverse analytical finding. US athletes should be particularly aware of Eldepryl (deprenyl or selegiline), Didrex (benzphetamine) and Gewodin (famprofazone, a nonsteroidal anti-inflammatory from Germany), which are metabolized to amphetamines. Several other drugs that metabolize to amphetamines are not available in the United States.

3.4 Use of injected epinephrine

Epinephrine (adrenaline) is prohibited in-competition only. If an athlete has an allergy which may produce an allergic reaction that is dangerous to health and requires that an epinephrine injector be carried, the athlete should carry the injector and take the medication as needed for an emergency. If an athlete is at a competition and uses the epinephrine for a medical emergency, or has used the epinephrine within a short period in advance of the competition, an emergency request for a TUE, as described under Section 4.7 of Reference 4, should be completed and submitted as soon as possible to the relevant anti-doping organization. The Emergency TUE must contain a full description of the medical situation that required the prohibited substance(s), all medications administered (including corticosteroids or other pharmaceuticals), the dosages and length of treatment. Note: In the review of an Emergency TUE request the committee is generally making the decision after the fact.

3.5 Over-the-counter products containing stimulants

Prohibited stimulants are sometimes present in over-the-counter substances such as cold medications, dietary supplements, diet aids and headache remedies

(Table 7.2). This is less of an issue than in the past because pseudoephedrine is now allowed in sport by the List; however, because of the methamphetamine production crisis in the United States President G.W. Bush signed the "Combat the Methamphetamine Epidemic Act of 2005" into law on March 9, 2006. This placed controls on the sale of chemical precursors of methamphetamine, such as pseudoephedrine.[11] Retail outlets must limit purchasers to 3.6 g of pseudoephedrine per day and to 9 g of the drug per 30-day day period. Mail service companies can sell no more than 7.5 g of pseudoephedrine in any form to an individual in any 30-day period and must confirm the purchaser's identity before shipping the product.

In addition, many states have enacted laws that are more rigid than the Federal Act of 2005. The individual state laws are summarized by the National Association of Chain Drug Stores.[12] In the event that the state law is more stringent, that law takes precedence over the federal law. In response, many pharmaceutical companies have reformulated over-the-counter medications to remove pseudoephedrine. In addition, the US Food and Drug Administration (FDA) has placed controls on the sales of ephedrine.[13]

There are still substances that require caution, such as the presence of L-methamphetamine in the Vicks Vapor Inhaler, and athletes must be very careful not to use preparations containing prohibited substances. Table 7.2 shows over-the-counter medications available in the United States that contain substances prohibited in-competition.

The stimulants are used for treatment of a number of medical conditions and can be useful away from a competition without being unfair within competition. Stimulants have only a short-term effect on performance, and if the drug is out of the body at the time of competition, there will not be an unfair advantage to the athlete. The athlete must be aware that the substance must be cleared from the blood and the urine, since urine is used for testing in the doping control program.

3.6 Modafinil

Modafinil[14] is a relatively new alertness-enhancing substance that was approved for use in the United States by the FDA in 1998 and is indicated to improve wakefulness in cases of narcolepsy, obstructive sleep apnea and shift work.[15]

Table 7.2 Over-the-counter medications that contain substances prohibited in-competition

Epinephrine	Ephedrine
MicroNefrin (solution for inhalation)	Mini Two-Way Action tablets
	Primatene tablets
Nephron (solution for inhalation)	Dynafed asthma relief tablets
S2 (solution for inhalation)	Bronkaid dual action tablets
Epinephrine mist (aerosol)	Ephedrine sulfate (tablets/capsules)
Primatene mist (aerosol)	Pretz-D nasal spray

Modafinil is prohibited as a stimulant by WADA and hit the world stage in 2003 when the investigation of the Bay Area Laboratory Cooperative (BALCO) found that elite athletes were being systematically doped with "undetectable" performance-enhancing substances to maximize benefit while reducing the possibility of detection. A USADA press release[16] summarizes the involvement of athletes in the use of modafinil. Modafinil improves alertness without the well-documented side effects of the central nervous stimulants such as methylphenidate[17] and amphetamine.[18]

La Garde *et al.*[19] found that modafinil reduced the frequency of involuntary microsleep episodes and kept subjects alert and maintained cognitive performance during 60 hours of sleep deprivation. Other studies have shown similar effects.[20–22] Caldwell[23] and Wesensten[24] have investigated the use of modafinil for wakefulness and sustained performance in the military environment. There appear to be benefits to the use of the drug; however, there are negative aspects, such as disruption of sleep following extended performance, that remain to be investigated.

3.7 Ephedrine

Ephedrine is prohibited in sport; however, the use of "ergogenic" aids has long been reported and is a practice that is continued today, to a large degree the result of advertising that promises enhanced performance in any number of areas. The supplement industry has been and continues to be full of charlatans who are very willing to advertise their products as containing unique ingredients that will bring performance enhancement in any number of areas, including muscle growth, sexual performance, endurance and mood. Unfortunately, the marketing of such products largely depends on emotional appeal and there are few scientific data to support such claims.

Ephedra is a genus of plant that consists of at least 40 species that can be found in Europe, North and South America, and Asia. *Ephedra* produces ephedrine and related alkaloids such as pseudoephedrine, norephedrine and norpseudoephedrine.[25] Ephedrine functions as a powerful agonist of both α- and β-adrenoceptors and acts as a sympathomimetic agent (mimicking the effects of adrenaline), working indirectly through this pathway by stimulating the release of norepinephrine from the adrenal medulla.[25] Although ephedrine and its related compounds have legitimate uses as a treatment for conditions such as asthma, bronchial constriction and hypotension, the abuse of the alkaloids by athletes and dieters has resulted in the controls mentioned earlier. In addition to the known physiological effects and apparent risks of this herbal supplement, there is only limited evidence that ephedrine will create the positive effects desired by the users.[26] As dietary supplements and ergogenic substances, ephedrine and its related alkaloids have been listed on supplement labels with a variety of different names, including Ma Huang, *Ephedra sinica*, *Ephedra equisetina* and ephedrine. Many of the supplements contain or are augmented by a synthesized ephedrine rather than the ephedrine produced naturally by *Ephedra*.

In a summary of several articles related to the effect of ephedrine on physical performance, Bucci[27] concludes that ephedrine alkaloids alone at concentrations greater than those found in the herbal extract did not enhance physical performance. The positive effects of ephedrine are, then, the effects of stimulation of the central nervous system (CNS) and are related to alertness and responsiveness (arousal). Combining ephedrine with caffeine has been found to significantly improve time to exhaustion in high-intensity exercise in a study of eight male subjects.[28] A similar study found that anaerobic performance was improved by the combination of substances and that ephedrine appeared to improve arousal and caffeine appeared to enhance muscle metabolism.[29] Ephedrine and related alkaloids have been found to produce adverse cardiovascular events.[30]

4 Beta-2 agonists (prohibited list – category S3)

All beta-2 agonists including their D- and L-isomers are prohibited.

As an exception, formoterol, salbutamol, salmeterol and terbutaline when administered by inhalation, require an Abbreviated Therapeutic Use Exemption.

Despite the granting of any form of Therapeutic Use Exemption, a concentration of salbutamol (free plus glucuronide) greater than 1000 ng/mL will be considered an *Adverse Analytical Finding* unless the *Athlete* proves that the abnormal result was the consequence of the therapeutic use of inhaled salbutamol.

4.1 Beta-2 agonists as stimulants

The choice of medications in the treatment of asthma and respiratory ailments has traditionally posed a challenge in sport. The β_2-agonists (stimulants) play a role in bronchodilation by interacting with the β_2-adrenoceptors. As a result, they are commonly used in sport by athletes with asthma or chronic obstructive pulmonary disease to relax the bronchial smooth muscle. The β_2-agonists are primarily used in treatment today by inhalation, in order to reduce the dosage, and are used as required to control asthma. The relative specificity of these medications and the lower dosages in use by inhalation reduce the overall stimulatory effect that would result from the use of nonselective β-agonists.[31] Many commonly prescribed β_2-agonists are powerful stimulants and may also possess anabolic properties, especially when taken orally or by injection. The β_2-agonists are widely used in sport, and in 2005 WADA received 609 adverse analytical reports (Table 7.3).[6]

Formoterol, salbutamol, salmeterol and terbutaline, though prohibited, can be used by inhalation if the appropriate anti-doping organization receives notification that the drug is being used (see Table 7.4 for examples of permitted brands). This notification is by the Abbreviated Therapeutic Use Exemption (TUE) form.[4] In the case of salbutamol (known in the United States as

Table 7.3 WADA adverse analytical findings for β_2 agonists

S3: β_2 Agonist	Occurrences	Percentage within drug class
Salbutamol	357	58.6
Terbutaline	171	28.1
Clenbuterol	52	8.5
Formoterol	18	3.0
Salmeterol	4	0.7
Reproterol	4	0.7
Fenoterol	3	0.5
Total[a]	**609**	

a Results for formoterol, salbutamol, salmeterol and terbutaline may correspond to administration by aerosol, which is permitted with certain restrictions as described in the Prohibited List. In addition, some adverse analytical findings correspond to multiple measurements on the same athlete.

Table 7.4 Examples of β_2 agonists permitted by Abbreviated TUE

Generic name	Pharmaceutical preparation
Formoterol, arformoterol, Salbutamol	Foradil, Brovana Albuterol (Albuterol HFA, Proventil, Proventil HFA, Ventolin, Ventolin HFA, Proair); levalbuterol (Xopenex, Xopenex HFA); Combivent and Duoneb (albuterol + ipratropium)
Salmeterol	Serevent, Advair and Advair HFA (salmeterol + fluticasone)
Terbutaline	Brethaire

albuterol), a concentration in the urine that is greater than 1000 ng/mL is an adverse analytical finding even if an Abbreviated TUE has been filed. There are no concentration limits on the other β_2-agonists that can be used with the Abbreviated TUE. Currently, many IFs require documentation such as medical records or pulmonary function tests to accompany an Abbreviated TUE for β_2-agonists for acceptance of the notification. It is the responsibility of the athlete to know the sport's IF requirements. The use of any β_2-agonist other than the four stated exceptions requires the submission and approval of a Standard TUE; the use of any of the four β_2-agonist exceptions listed above by a mode of administration other than inhalation requires that a Standard TUE be submitted and approved.

5 Specified substances

The List identifies substances which are particularly susceptible to unintentional anti-doping rule violations because of their general availability in prescription or over-the-counter pharmaceuticals and which are less likely to be used as doping agents. These are identified as "specified substances," and a doping violation involving a specified substance may result in a reduced sanction if the "Athlete can establish that the Use of such a specified substance was not intended to enhance sport performance." The "Specified Substances" as of 1 January 2008[5] are:

- All inhaled Beta-2 agonists, except salbutamol (free plus glucuronide) greater than 1000 ng/mL and clenbuterol (listed under S1.2: Other Anabolic Agents);
- Alpha-reductase inhibitors, probenecid;
- Cathine, cropropamide, crotetamide, ephedrine, etamivan, famprofazone, heptaminol, isometheptene, levmethamfetamine, meclofenoxate, p-methylamphetamine, methylephedrine, nikethamide, norfenefrine, octopamine, ortetamine, oxilofrine, phenpromethamine, propylhexedrine, selegiline, sibutramine, tuaminoheptane and any other stimulant not expressly listed under section S6 for which the Athlete establishes that it fulfils the conditions described in section S6;
- Cannabinoids;
- All Glucocorticosteroids;
- *Alcohol;*
- *All Beta Blockers.*

6 Diuretics and other masking agents (prohibited list – category S5)

Masking agents are prohibited. They include:
Diuretics*, epitestosterone, probenecid, alpha-reductase inhibitors (e.g. **finasteride, dutasteride), plasma expanders** (e.g. **albumin, dextran, hydroxyethyl starch)** and other substances with similar biological effect(s).
Diuretics include:
Acetazolamide, amiloride, bumetanide, canrenone, chlorthalidone, etacrynic acid, furosemide, indapamide, metolazone, spironolactone, thiazides (e.g. **bendroflumethiazide, chlorothiazide, hydrochlorothiazide), triamterene**, and other substances with a similar chemical structure or similar biological effect(s) (except for drosperinone, which is not prohibited).
A Therapeutic Use Exemption is not valid if an *Athlete*'s urine contains a diuretic in association with threshold or sub-threshold levels of a *Prohibited Substance*(s).

6.1 Status of diuretics and masking agents in sport

Masking agents are substances or methods that are used to prevent the detection of other substances or methods used by an athlete for doping. Diuretics

Table 7.5 WADA adverse analytical findings for diuretics, 2005

S5: Diuretics and other masking agents	Occurrences	Percentage within drug class
Furosemide	91	37.0
Hydrochlorothiazide	67	27.2
Finasteride	28	11.4
Canrenone	14	5.7
Amiloride	10	4.1
Triamterene	9	3.7
Acetazolamide	6	2.4
Epitestosterone	5	2.0
Bendroflumethazide	5	2.0
Indapamide	4	1.6
Clorothiazide	3	1.2
Spironolactone	1	0.4
Piretanide	1	0.4
Chlortalidone	1	0.4
Bumetanide	1	0.4
Total[a]	**246**	

a Some adverse analytical findings may correspond to multiple findings on the same athlete.

(Table 7.5)[6] are considered to be one type of masking agent and are drugs that help the body to eliminate fluids (water and salts) by increasing the rate of urine formation. Although diuretics, under strict medical supervision, have important therapeutic uses for the elimination of excess fluid from the body for certain diseases and for management of high blood pressure, they are prohibited both in- and out-of-competition. Diuretics may be abused by athletes to reduce weight quickly in sports where weight categories are involved, and/or to produce a more rapid excretion of urine to reduce the concentration of prohibited substances in the urine in an attempt to escape detection.

Drastic reduction of weight in sport cannot be medically justified. The potential for serious side effects such as dehydration, muscle cramps, volume depletion, drop in blood pressure and severe electrolyte imbalance exists. Deliberate attempts to reduce weight artificially, in order to compete in lower weight classes or to dilute urine, constitutes clear manipulation, which is ethically unacceptable. Diuretics promote the excretion of water and electrolytes by the kidneys. They are used in the treatment of heart failure or in hepatic, renal or pulmonary disease when salt and water retention has resulted in edema or ascites. Diuretics are also used, either alone or in association with other drugs, in the treatment of hypertension, although the mechanism for their antihypertensive effect is poorly understood. Taken without medical supervision, diuretics can result in potassium depletion and death.

The principal groups of diuretics are as follows:[32]

- Carbonic anhydrase inhibitors are weak diuretics and are used mainly to reduce elevated intra-ocular pressure. Examples of this group of diuretics are acetazolamide, dorzolamide and methazolamide.

- "Loop" or "high-ceiling" diuretics produce an intense, dose-dependent diuresis of relatively short duration. Examples of this group of diuretics are etacrynic acid and furosemide.
- Osmotic diuretics raise the osmolality of plasma and renal tubular fluid. They are used to reduce or prevent cerebral oedema, to reduce raised intraocular pressure and in acute renal failure. Examples of this group of diuretics are isosorbide and mannitol.
- Potassium-sparing diuretics have a relatively weak diuretic effect and are normally used in conjunction with thiazide or loop diuretics. Examples are amiloride, canrenone, eplerenone, spironolactone and triamterene. These diuretics are aldosterone antagonists and are particularly used in conditions where aldosterone contributes to the pathophysiology.
- Thiazides (benzothiadiazines), such as bendroflumethiazide and hydrochlorothiazide, and certain other compounds, such as metolazone, with structural similarities to the thiazides, inhibit sodium and chloride reabsorption in the kidney tubules and produce a corresponding increase in potassium excretion.

If an athlete has a legitimate medical need for a diuretic, they may, with certain restrictions, apply for a Standard TUE. In addition to diuretics, there are other means to attempt masking of doping. Examples would be an attempt to change the pH of the urine to enhance excretion of a doping substance, the use of substances such as probenecid to reduce renal excretion of doping substances, use of epitestosterone to minimize the possibility of detection of doping with testosterone by keeping the T/E ratio below the threshold of 4, the addition of chemicals or other contaminants to the actual specimen following collection (sample tampering), substitution of a specimen provided for doping controls, or the destruction of collection documents. Basically, masking is the use of a specific substance or a method to prevent anti-doping authorities from otherwise detecting doping. Any attempt to cover doping is prohibited either under this category of substances or under the M2 category of the List, which prohibits methods of manipulation.

7 Summary

The World Anti-Doping Program is made up of the Code, which is a policy document, and various international standards, which include a list of prohibited substances and methods, and the procedures for requests for a TUE for the legitimate medical use of an otherwise prohibited substance. Two significant points are as follows:

1   A prohibited substance or prohibited method does not have to enhance performance to be prohibited. It is enough that the prohibited substance or prohibited method was present in the sample, or attempted to be used, for a doping violation to have occurred.

2   The presence of a prohibited substance in an athlete's urine (or blood, when applicable) constitutes an offense, regardless of the manner in which the prohibited substance came to be in the athlete's system.

Amphetamines and the related CNS stimulants ephedrine and modafinil are prohibited in-competition; however, the stimulants may be used out-of-competition if the stimulant and any metabolites are cleared from the body (including urine) by the time an in-competition test is administered. The use of any stimulant (such as amphetamine or methylphenidate) in-competition requires that a Standard TUE be submitted and approved prior to the use of the drug in-competition. A number of the stimulants are considered "specified substances," which in certain conditions allows that a reduced sanction be considered if a doping violation has occurred.

β_2-agonists are prohibited both in- and out-of-competition with the exception that four drugs of the class may be used if an Abbreviated TUE is properly completed and filed. The β_2-agonists are stimulants and may have anabolic activity. β_2-agonists are also considered to be "specified substances," so that a reduced sanction may be considered if a doping violation has occurred. The use of any β_2-agonists (other than the four exceptions) requires that a Standard TUE be submitted and approved prior to the use in sport either in- or out-of-competition. The presence of salbutamol in the urine at a concentration greater than 1000 ng/mL may be a doping violation even if an Abbreviated TUE has been properly filed.

Diuretics may be used to make weight or to mask the use of other prohibited substances by increasing the rate of elimination from the body. Both diuretics and other masking agents are prohibited both in- and out-of-competition, but continue to be abused in sport and result in doping violations. The use of any of the diuretics or masking agents in sport for legitimate medical purposes must be covered by an approved Standard TUE. The diuretics are not on the "Specified Substance" list.

Finasteride to enhance hair growth and dutasteride for the treatment of benign prostatic hypertrophy are masking agents for certain anabolic steroids and are prohibited. Their use in sport requires an approved Standard TUE, although these medications are considered to be "specified substances."

8 Acknowledgments

I should like to thank Drs Larry Bowers and Jeffery Podraza for their constructive comments on this chapter and Ms Carla O'Connell and Ms Camila Zardo for editorial and preparation assistance. Despite the assistance, I must accept responsibility for any errors or misrepresentations which may be included in the writing. The opinions expressed herein are those of the author and do not represent any official position or policy of USADA. Please note that the international standard for TUEs and the list are currently being updated. Please check those specific documents for rules that will apply 1 January 2009.

9 References

1 Aziz, RA. History of drugs in sport, WADA Asia Education Symposium. Available from http://www.wada-ama.org/rtecontent/document/history_of_doping_dr_ramlan_abdul_aziz.pdf (accessed February 28, 2007).

2 Fotheringham W. *Put me back on my bike: in search of Tom Simpson*. London: Yellow Jersey Press, 2002.

3 World Anti-Doping Agency. The World Anti-Doping Code, Version 3. Available, from: http://www.wada-ama.org/rtecontent/document/code_v3.pdf (accessed January 12, 2007).

4 World Anti-Doping Agency. International Standard for Therapeutic Use Exemptions. Available from http://www.wada-ama.org/rtecontent/document/international_standard.pdf (accessed January 12, 2007).

5 World Anti-Doping Agency, 2008 Prohibited List, International Standard. Available from http://www.wada-ama.org/rtecontent/document/2008_List_En.pdf (accessed November 4, 2007).

6 World Anti-Doping Agency, 2006 Statistical Report, Table G. Available, from http://www.wada-ama.org/rtecontent/document/labstats_2005.pdf (accessed November 6, 2007).

7 Department of Justice, Drug Enforcement Agency: General Reference for Drug Scheduling. Available from http://www.usdoj.gov/dea/pubs/scheduling.html (accessed October 8, 2007).

8 *Martindale 2005: The Complete Drug Reference*, 34th ed. Ed. Sweetman SC. London: Pharmaceutical Press, 2005; 852–3.

9 Jacobs M. Fatal amphetamine-associated cardiotoxicity and its medicolegal implications. *American Journal of Forensic Medicine and Pathology*. 2006; 27: 156–60.

10 US Food and Drug Administration. FDA directs ADHD drug manufacturers to notify patients about cardiovascular adverse events and psychiatric adverse events. *FDA News*, February 21, 2007. Available from http://www.fda.gov/bbs/topics/news/2007, new01568.html (accessed April 9, 2007).

11 House Report 109–333 – USA PATRIOT Improvement and Reauthorization Act of 2005. Available from http://thomas.loc.gov/cgi-bin/cpquery/?&dbname=cp109 &sid=cp109djs6R&refer=&r_n=hr333.109&item=&sel=TOC_358801&%3e (accessed November 6, 2007).

12 National Association of Chain Drug Stores. Available from http://www.nacds.org/wmspage.cfm?parm1=3814 (accessed November 6, 2007).

13 Federal Register, February 6, 2004. DHHS, FDA, 21 CFR Part 119. Final rule declaring dietary supplements containing ephedrine alkaloids adulterated because they present an unreasonable risk. Available from http://www.fda.gov/OHRMS/DOCKETS/98fr/1995n-0304-nfr0001.pdf (accessed October 8, 2007).

14 Modafinil, sold as Provigil, prescription only, Cephalon, Inc., West Chester, PA 19380.

15 *Physicians' Desk Reference*, 61st ed. Ed. PDR. Montvale, NJ: Thomson PDR, 2007; 988–93.

16 USADA press release, Track and Field athletes Montgomery and Gaines receive suspensions for doping violations. December 13, 2005. Available from http://www.usantidoping.org/resources/press/press_archive.aspx (accessed September 19, 2007).

17 Kollins S, MacDonald E, Rush C. Assessing the abuse potential of methylphenidate in nonhuman and human subjects: a review. *Pharmacology Biochemistry and Behavior* 68: 611–27.

18 Baselt, R. *Disposition of toxic drugs and chemicals in man*, 6th ed. Foster City, CA: Biomedical Publications, 2000; 64–6.

19 La Garde D, Batejat D, Van Beers P, Sarafian D, Pradella S. Interest of modafinil, a new psychostimulant, during a sixty-hour sleep deprivation experiment. *Fundamental Clinical Pharmacology*. 1995; 9: 271–9.

20 Pigeau R, Naitsh P, Buguet A, McCann C. Modafinil, d-amphetamine, and placebo during 64 hours of sustained mental work 1. Effects on mood, fatigue, cognitive performance, and body temperature. *Journal of Sleep Research*. 1995; 4: 212–28.

21 Wesensten N, Belenky G, Kautz MA, Thorne D, Balkin TJ. Sustaining cognitive performance during sleep deprivation: relative efficacy of modafinil (100, 200, and 400 mg) versus caffeine. *Psychopharmacology*. 2002; 159: 238–47.

22 Turner DC, Robbins TW, Clark L, Aron AR, Dowson J, Sahakian BJ. Cognitive enhancing effects of modafinil in healthy volunteers. *Psychopharmacology*. 2003; 165: 260–9.

23 Caldwell JA Jr, Caldwell JL, Smythe NK III, Hall KK. 2000 A double-blind, placebo-controlled investigation of the efficacy of modafinil for sustaining the alertness and performance of aviators: a helicopter simulator study. *Psychopharmacology*. 2000: 150: 272–82.

24 Wesensten N. Effects of modafinil on cognitive performance and alertness during sleep deprivation. *Current Pharmaceutical Design*. 2006; 12(20): 2457–71.

25 Bruneton J. Phenethylamines. In: *Pharmacognosy, phytochemistry, medicinal plants*, Part 4: Alkaloids: phenethylamines. Paris: Lavoisier, 1995; 712–13.

26 Shekelle PG, Hardy ML, Morton SC, Maglione M, Suttorp M, Roth E, Jungvig L, Mojica WA, Gagné J, Rhodes S, McKinnon E. Ephedra and ephedrine for weight loss and athletic performance enhancement: clinical efficacy and side effects. Evidence Report/Technology Assessment No. 76 (prepared by Southern California Evidence-Based Practice Center, RAND, under contract 290–97–0001, Task Order No. 9) AHRQ Publication 03-E022. Rockville, MD: Agency for Healthcare Research and Quality.

27 Bucci L. Selected herbals and human exercise performance. *American Journal of Clinical Nutrition*. 1998; 72(Suppl): 624–36.

28 Bell D, Jacobs I, Ameccnik J. Effects of caffeine, ephedrine, and their combination on time to exhaustion during high-intensity exercise. *European Journal of Applied Physiology*. 1998; 77: 427–33.

29 Bell D, Jacobs I, Ellerington K. Effects of caffeine and ephedrine ingestion on anaerobic exercise performance. *Medicine and Science in Sports and Exercise*. 2001; 33: 1399–403.

30 Haller C, Benowitz N. Adverse cardiovascular and central nervous system events associated with dietary supplements containing ephedra alkaloids. *New England Journal of Medicine*. 2000; 343: 1833–8.

31 *Martindale 2005: The Complete Drug Reference*, 34th ed. Ed. Sweetman SC. London: Pharmaceutical Press, 2005; 777.

32 *Martindale 2005: The Complete Drug Reference*, 34th ed. Ed. Sweetman SC. London: Pharmaceutical Press, 2005; 811.

8 Erythropoietin doping

Detection in urine

Françoise Lasne

1 Introduction

Erythropoietin (EPO) is better known by the public for its use in doping than as a medication. A good number of scandals have erupted regarding its use in sports, and these constitute just a shadow of its use as a doping agent. It is true that the biological effects of this hormone, which is normally synthesized in the kidney by the peritubular cells of the proximal tubule, have a well-known impact on aerobic power and therefore upon the athlete's capacity for endurance. By stimulating the production of red blood cells by the bone marrow, EPO improves the transport of oxygen to muscles.

EPO was placed on the list of forbidden substances in 1990 by the International Olympic Committee, but it was only in 2000 during the Olympic Games in Sydney that this hormone became the subject of anti-doping testing, using both an indirect blood test and a direct urine test. The indirect test aimed to establish stimulation of erythropoiesis induced by this hormone, while the direct test rested on the demonstration of the presence of the doping agent in the urine. Thus, the indirect test suggested the establishment of a score based on the combination of values of five parameters: hematocrit (Hct), reticulocyte hematocrit (Ret Hct), percentage of macrocytes (%macro), serum EPO, and soluble receptors of transferrin (sTfr), to reveal a recent administration of EPO (ON-model). A second score using three of the above parameters (Hct, Ret Hct and serum EPO) was intended to detect an earlier administration of this hormone (OFF-model).[1] The aim of the direct test was to demonstrate the exogenous origin of the EPO present in the urine of subjects treated by this hormone. Indeed, since a part of the EPO created by the organism is present in urine, it was imperative to differentiate this endogenous EPO ("natural") from that administered in the case of doping.

In 2002, the direct urine test was adopted for anti-doping control, and the indirect blood test (and its variations) is currently used by certain sport federations for targeting the athletes who will be subject to a urine test.

This chapter is concerned with the direct detection of EPO in urine.

2 Principle of the test

At the time of the development of the direct urine test, two pharmaceutical specialties had already been proposed for the treatment of certain forms of anemia (in particular, that linked to a chronic renal insufficiency), and these were liable to be utilized for doping: the epoetins alfa and beta patented by Amgen and Genetics Institute, respectively. These two hormones are both recombinant proteins – that is to say, produced by host cells whose DNA has been modified by genetic recombination to introduce the gene of human EPO. In both cases, CHO (Chinese hamster ovary) cells were used as host cell system. The resulting recombinant EPO has a structure very close to that of human urinary EPO. Both natural urinary and recombinant hormones are a 165 amino acid glycoprotein with three N-linked (Asp-24, -38, and -83) and one O-linked (Ser-126) oligosaccharide side chains. As yet, antibodies specific to the natural or recombinant form do not exist. Immunoassay of this hormone in blood or urine shows no distinction between the natural or recombinant hormone, so it is of no use in identifying its origin.

The differentiation between these kinds of EPO rests on the analysis of their isoelectric profiles. The peptide backbone of these molecules is identical since in both cases it is encoded by the gene of human EPO. However, during and after its synthesis this polypeptide undergoes different post-translational modifications. Thus, an important glycosylation causes about 40 percent of the molecule of EPO to be constituted of three complex type N-glycans and one mucin type O-glycan. Other post-translational modifications, little known for EPO, can affect the peptide and/or the polysaccharide parts of a glycoprotein (phosphorylation, sulfation, etc.). None of these modifications is under the direct control of the gene encoding the polypeptide moiety; rather, they depend on the enzymatic equipment of the cell making the synthesis. They are not exactly identical for all of the molecules of a given protein. This is one of multiple mechanisms explaining the general phenomenon of "microheterogeneity" of proteins.

Some of these post-translational modifications affect the electrical charge of the molecule. This is why it is possible to have a partial indication (only detecting the differences playing upon the electrical charge) of microhetero- geneity when using a charge-based separation method such as isoelectric focusing (IEF). This indication is revealed by the presence of several isoforms (molecular forms of the same protein showing differences in electrical charges) constituting the isoelectric pattern of the protein. Natural EPO is synthesized by human kidney cells in a living organism whereas recombinant EPO is obtained from cultured CHO cells. The starting hypothesis for the urine test was that some of the post-translational modifications affecting these hormones would present differences relating to the species, to the tissue type and to the environmental conditions of the cells involved in the synthesis. In this case, these differences would very likely be indicated by the isoelectric patterns of these hormones.

3 Method

The method includes three steps. Only the principle of these steps and some comments explaining the usefulness of particular points can be covered here. For more technical details, see Lasne *et al.*[2] The scope of the first step is to concentrate urine with EPO, whose starting level is usually only a few international units per liter (IU/L), corresponding to a couple of tens of nanograms per liter. The second step is the separation of the EPO isoforms. The last step is the detection of these isoforms that constitute the isoelectric pattern of the hormone.

3.1 First step: concentration

After adjustment of the pH to 7.4 and addition of an anti-protease cocktail, 18 mL of previously microfiltered urine is concentrated by ultrafiltration. Since different enzymes are present in urine, it is essential to prevent the action of proteases that could degrade EPO during a concentration process. Centrifugal filter devices with a molecular weight cutoff (MWCO) of 30 kDa are used to finally obtain a retentate of about 20–50 µL. Although the cutoff of 30 kD is very close to the molecular mass of EPO (34 kD), the latter is totally retained in the retentate. This process allows molecules of low molecular weight to be eliminated in the filtrate. This filtrate can be used for other anti-doping analysis. During this step, the retentates are washed (diafiltration) with a buffer suitable for the next step. The retentates are assayed for their EPO level by enzyme-linked immunosorbent assay (ELISA) and diluted or not according to this level just before the second step.

3.2 Second step: isoelectric focusing (IEF)

The retentates from the ultrafiltration are submitted to IEF in a polyacrylamide gel containing 7M urea, pH gradient 2–6. At this stage, the different proteins present in the retentate are separated according to their pI and each one is separated into its constituent isoforms. Before being put on to the gel, the different retentates are heated to 80 °C for 2 minutes. This treatment does not affect EPO[3] but allows the denaturing of the acidic proteases that could be reactivated by the acidic conditions of the IEF. Indeed, without heating, EPO completely disappears during IEF.

3.3 Third step: detection of the EPO isoelectric profiles

At the end of the IEF, the gel is submitted to immunoblotting using a primary anti-human EPO antibody (monoclonal AE7A5) and a secondary biotinylated goat anti-mouse immunoglobulin G (IgG) antibody in order to specifically detect the EPO isoforms by way of a chemiluminescence reaction.

When the test was developed, it was obvious that the usual immunoblotting method did not function. Indeed, the isoforms of EPO are "drowned"

among those of the different proteins present in the retentate. Nonspecific interactions occurred between some of these proteins and the secondary antibody,
and this prevented any specific detection of EPO. This problem was undoubt-
edly the most difficult to resolve, and it required the development of a new
method of immunoblotting called "double blotting" (DB).[4,5] In this procedure,
the proteins are transferred from the IEF gel to a first polyvinylidene fluoride
(PVDF) blotting membrane called the "blotting membrane" (B membrane),
which, after saturation, is incubated with the primary anti-EPO antibodies.
A second PVDF membrane called the "double blotting membrane" (DB
membrane) is layered onto the B membrane (with an intermediate membrane
between them) in acidic conditions. The intermediate membrane has no affinity
for the proteins. The membranes are placed in a semi-dry blotting apparatus in
such a way that the DB membrane is facing the cathode (Figure 8.1A). Owing to
the acidic conditions, the primary antibody is desorbed from EPO and, having a
positive charge, is transferred by the electrical field through the intermediate
membrane onto the DB membrane. At the end of this process, all the interfering
proteins and the EPO itself are retained on the B membrane since the
acidity does not affect their hydrophobic interactions with this membrane.
The anti-EPO antibodies are thus isolated on a "clean" membrane (the DB
membrane), which can then be used for incubation with the secondary antibodies without any risk of a nonspecific adsorption (Figure 8.1B). Note that at the
end of the DB process, the B membrane can be kept in a buffer to be probed
again with a primary antibody (the same as or different from the first time).

After treatment with the secondary biotinylated antibodies, the DB
membrane is incubated with streptavidine–peroxydase complexes and a
chemiluminescent substrate. Light emission is detected by a charge-coupled
device (CCD) camera. The result of the test is thus an image of the isoelectric
pattern of EPO present in a urine sample.

4 Results

4.1 Images of EPO isoelectric patterns

As is shown in Figure 8.2, the recombinant epoetins alfa and beta appear to be
composed of six and seven isoforms respectively, with pI in the range 4.4–5.1.

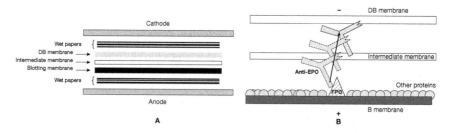

Figure 8.1 Double blotting. (A) Experimental set-up; (B) principle of the method.

The pattern of another recombinant EPO, darbepoietin alfa or NESP (Novel Erythopoiesis-Stimulating Protein) from Amgen, has been included in this figure because, with BRP (Biological Reference Preparation, constituted of an equimolecular mixture of epoetins alfa and beta), it establishes guiding marks on the image that permit the characterization of the EPO profiles tested. Thus, numbers and letters have been assigned to the different bands composing a pattern, a zone called the "basic area" has been defined by the position of BRP, and an "acidic area" by that of NESP.

Natural urinary EPO (here, purified as a preliminary) is more heterogeneous, because it can be composed of up to 16 isoforms extending on a pH gradient from 3.7 to 5.1. If some of its isoforms coincide with those of epoetins alfa and beta and of NESP, its pattern is clearly different from that of these recombinant hormones, since the most intense of its isoforms are situated in a zone called the "endogenous area" (between the basic and the acidic areas). Even if this pattern presents variations from one individual to another, or in some cases from one sample to another in the same individual (see the case of "effort urine", p. 116), it is the basis of every urinary profile in the absence of doping.

When recombinant EPO is administered, part of the dose injected is found in the urine without great changes in its isoelectric pattern. Only a slight acidification of this pattern is observed, so that the presence of recombinant EPO in the urine is obvious. In some cases, the pattern of the eliminated recombinant product completely replaces that of the endogenous EPO. This may be explained by the dilution of the natural hormone by its recombinant analogue, and/or by the negative feedback induced by the increased oxygenation due to a higher level of red blood cells. In other cases, the pattern shows the presence in urine of both endogenous and recombinant EPO hormones.

The presence of recombinant EPO is clearly shown by the image of the isoelectric pattern observed in a urine sample. Nevertheless, this first visual interpretation is then completed by a quantification of the isoforms. The profile obtained has to meet criteria for positivity in an objective way to demonstrate the presence of recombinant EPO.

4.2 Interpretation of results: the criteria for positivity

The intensities of luminescence of the isoforms are estimated using a software program for integration of the numerical data from the camera. Different programs can be used. One of them, "GASepo," has been developed by the anti-doping laboratory in Vienna especially for EPO analysis.[6] The images of the different EPO patterns are thus converted into profiles.

For this, a densitometer window is positioned on each lane, analyzed using reference marks provided by the patterns of BRP and NESP having migrated on the same IEF gel. The relative intensities of the bands situated inside this window are then examined according to preestablished criteria for positivity. The specificity of these criteria has been tested on control populations,

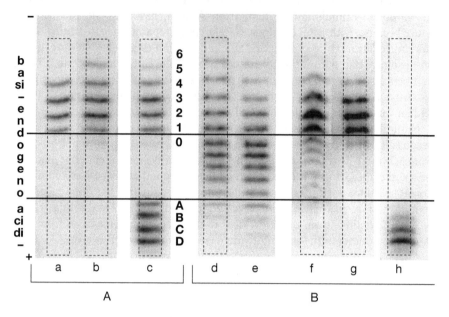

Figure 8.2 Isoelectric patterns of erythropoietin (EPO). (A) Images obtained from pure products: epoetin alfa (a), epoetin beta (b), a mixture of BRP (top) and NESP (bottom) used as references to assign band numbers to the different lanes (c). (B) Urine samples showing the presence of natural endogenous urinary EPO (d, e) or recombinant hormones epoetin alfa or beta (f, g) and NESP (h). Note the presence of both natural and recombinant EPO in (f). The dotted boxes correspond to the densitometer windows.

permitting to exclude, with a negligible risk of error, the possibility of a "false positive."

Different criteria for positivity have been successively proposed. Historically, the "percentage of basic isoforms" (the sum of the relative intensities located in the basic area of a profile) was first used (in 2000). A threshold value of 80 percent was required, beyond which the presence of recombinant EPO was declared.

This criterion, subsequently found to be restricted to cases with a quasi-total absence of natural endogenous EPO in the profile, was then replaced by criteria that permitted the detection of recombinant EPO in the presence of endogenous hormone. To sum up, the presence of recombinant EPO was reported if isoforms 1 and 2 or 2 and 3 were the most intense of the profile (TD2004EPO and TD20007EPO documents from World Anti-Doping Agency). Better performance criteria are required to detect the use of low doses of EPO by athletes. Interpretation of isoelectric profiles by discriminant analysis has been proposed, and proved to be the most sensitive method to detect low doses of recombinant EPO.[7]

5 Introduction of a purification step by immunoaffinity

Among the technical modifications developed since the original use of the test, the possibility of a purification step by immunoaffinity was introduced in the preparation step. This allows the extraction of EPO from the urinary matrix and is used in confirmation analysis of a sample if the electrophoretic migration has shown defects linked to a protein surcharge of the analyzed retentate. In this case, immunoaffinity clearly improves the quality of the images and thus facilitates their integration (Figure 8.3A).

On the other hand, some scientists have criticized the use of monoclonal AE7A5 antibody as primary antibody for the immunoblotting step. This antibody has been described as nonspecific for EPO and would recognize other proteins interfering in the final result of an anti-doping control. In fact, these assertions rely on incorrect extrapolations of observations made using totally different analytical methods (such as immunohistochemistry). In the analytical conditions of the test, the only protein other than EPO (identified as α_2 Zn glycoprotein by the Austrian anti-doping laboratory) that is recognized by this antibody is situated outside the densitometer window used for interpreting a profile and thus does not interfere in the result. This is reliably demonstrated by comparing the results obtained by including or not including the immunoaffinity step in the procedure. Indeed, the immunoaffinity step uses an anti-human EPO antibody (clone 9C21D11) that is different from the one used for immunoblotting (clone AE7A5). When the immunoaffinity step is included in the preparation step, the final image results from the use of both antibodies. In this case, as shown by Figure 8.3B, there is no change in the EPO pattern when compared to the profile obtained without immunoaffinity. This demonstrates that inside the densitometer window used to interpret a result, no protein interferes with the detection of EPO by the antibody AE7A5. As expected, the additional specificity brought by the immunoaffinity step makes disappear only the isoforms corresponding to α_2 Zn glycoprotein that is outside the densitometer window.

6 Possible modifications of EPO profiles

The urinary EPO profiles corresponding to natural hormone may in some cases present singularities that have been taken into account when rules were set for interpretation of results. Two kinds of circumstances are at the origin of these individual profiles.

6.1 Unstable urine samples

Different enzymes can be present in urine: proteases, glycosidases, sulfatases, neuraminidases, etc. For this reason, it is very important to protect EPO from the action of these enzymes during the phases of concentration by ultrafiltration and of IEF of the samples. Nonetheless, it can happen that enzymatic

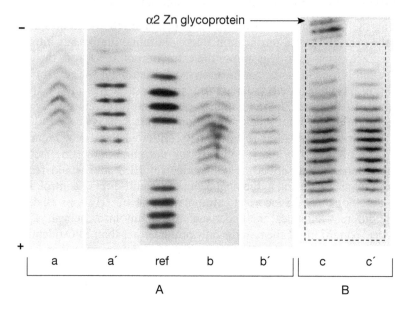

α2 Zn glycoprotein ⟶

a   a′   ref   b   b′   c   c′

A   B

Figure 8.3 Introduction of a purification step by immunoaffinity. (A) Improvement of the electrophoretic migration: two urine samples with a high protein content were analyzed without (a, b) and with (a′, b′) the immunoaffinity step. (B) Specificity of the EPO pattern inside the densitometer window: the same urine sample was analyzed without (c) and with (c′) the immunoaffinity step.

activity may have already altered the EPO by the time the sample reaches the lab. This has been observed essentially when the sample has travelled under poor conditions (too long a delay, or high ambient temperatures). When urine samples are obtained in the absence of any precautions for aseptic conditions, it seems that the enzymatic activity of the samples is linked to the proliferation of bacteria that develop during the transport.[8]

6.1.1 Consequences for the EPO profile

Three different cases may be observed. In the first case, ELISA indicates that the retentate obtained from ultrafiltration of urine in the preparative step of the test is devoid of EPO. This situation may, of course, correspond to a true low secretion and excretion of this hormone in urine. However, in some of these cases EPO is in fact digested by the proteases that are present in urine (in particular, acidic proteases). This situation results in a blank image when analyzed by IEF.

In the second case, ELISA indicates sufficient concentration of EPO in the retentate to be visualized by IEF. However, a blank image is obtained, as in the previous case. This discrepancy between ELISA and IEF will be explained shortly.

In the third case, the IEF reveals unusual patterns of EPO composed of isoforms located in the basic part of the pH gradient. However, these patterns are clearly different from those of urine samples positive for epoetin alfa or beta. Indeed, whereas the most intense bands are numbers 1, 2 or 3 in epoetin-positive cases, they are in a more basic position in active urine samples (Figure 8.4A). These basic bands in fact correspond to EPO isoforms shifted by the enzymatic removal of negative electrical charges. In this situation, it is thus impossible to know whether the EPO was initially natural or recombinant, and the result of the test is "unclassifiable result, degraded urine sample."

The second case described above (discrepancy between the ELISA result and the absence of an IEF image) corresponds to high shifting activity causing the EPO isoforms to be located outside the 2–6 pH gradient used for the analysis. When a broader pH gradient (2–8) is used, these shifted isoforms are detected (Figure 8.4B).

Whereas the first two cases give rise to an unambiguous EPO test result of "undetectable EPO," it is very important to differentiate the third case (shifting activity within the pH gradient 2–6) from a true positive case for epoetin. That is why a stability test in which the shifting activity of urine is tested toward recombinant EPO is systematically performed at the time of the confirmatory analysis of anti-doping control. For this, the tested urine sample is incubated with recombinant EPO (BRP and darbepoetin alfa) before IEF and double

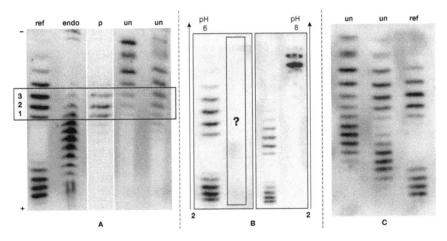

Figure 8.4 Unstable urine samples. (A) Unstable samples giving rise to shifted isoelectric patterns; note the different distribution of the basic bands in case of unstable urine samples (un) in comparison with cases positive for epoetin (p). (B) In spite of a sufficient EPO level in the retentate, no EPO bands are detected after isoelectric focusing in the usual pH gradient (2–6). These bands appear if the pH gradient is extended toward basic values (2–8). (C) Stability test: a clear shift of the references BRP and NESP (ref) is observed when incubated in unstable urine samples (un).

blotting of this hormone. Since the sample is directly submitted to IEF without any concentration by ultrafiltration, its endogenous EPO is not detected. The result permits the assessment of any shift in the position of the added recombinant EPO (Figure 8.4C). If any shift is observed, the sample is considered "unstable" and this rules out any interpretation of its own EPO pattern.

6.1.2 Frequency of unstable urine samples

Unstable urine samples are rare. Out of 577 samples analyzed in our laboratory in 2003, 8 gave rise to shifted EPO profiles and 8 to EPO profiles outside of the pH gradient 2–6. Because bacterial proliferation appeared to be implicated in the activity, 348 urine samples analyzed for EPO from January to August 2004 were submitted to direct microscopic examination. Since many of these samples had been frozen immediately after collection, only 56 of them presented bacterial proliferation. As can be seen in Figure 8.5, the proportion of samples with altered EPO was clearly greater in these 56 samples.

These observations point to the importance of preventing bacterial proliferation between collection and analysis of urine samples.

6.2 "Effort" profiles

"Effort" profiles are encountered more often than unstable urine samples. "Effort" profiles are observed in the case of certain urine samples taken after

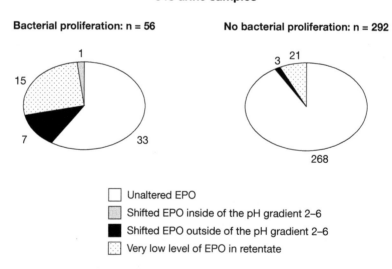

Figure 8.5 Results of EPO testing from January to August 2004 in the French anti-doping laboratory.

some types of strenuous physical exercise. Such profiles present an intensifica-
tion of the isoforms situated in the basic area, so that the whole profile seems
to be moved slightly toward the cathode (Figure 8.6).

Comparison of EPO profiles in serum and urine has shown that natural EPO is more acidic in urine (Figure 8.7), but the mechanism of this
acidification process remains unknown.[9,10] It is possible that the temporary
proteinuria (including a significant rise in the EPO level) occurring after
exercise exceeds the capacity of the mechanisms involved in the acidification
of EPO and thus gives rise to the more basic isoforms observed in "effort"
profiles.

The criteria for positivity have been elaborated, taking into account this
phenomenon, to distinguish between an effort profile and the presence of
epoietin alfa or beta.

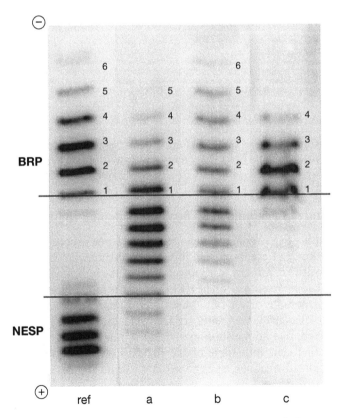

Figure 8.6 Effort profile. A typical aspect of the pattern as observed after some particularly strenuous physical exercise is shown in (b). For comparison, patterns
of typical endogenous urinary EPO (a) and epoetin alfa excreted in urine
(c) are shown.

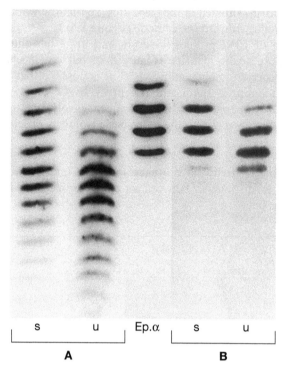

Figure 8.7 Comparison of serum and urine EPO. Both endogenous (A) and injected recombinant (B) EPO are more acidic in urine (U) than in serum (S). The pattern of the injected hormone, epoetin alfa, is shown for comparison (Ep. α).

7 The future of erythropoietin doping and doping control

Doping with EPO is going to change, and in some aspects is already changing. Three kinds of events explain this. First, athletes who cheat try to escape a possible positive control by using lower doses of the hormone. Second, the pharmaceutical companies develop new EPO products for treatment of patients that enrich the medicine chest of athletes too. Finally, genetic technologies are expected to change the very nature of medical treatments. It is now conceivable, and predicted, that administration of EPO will be replaced by introducing the corresponding gene into some of the patient's own cells. While the two first points are already realities, let us hope that the third still lies in the future.

7.1 Low doses of recombinant human EPO

The doses in clinical practice are adjusted by supervision of hemoglobin and/or hematocrit values in the patient and are different depending on the nature of the disease and the responsiveness of the patient. Unnecessary administration of recombinant human EPO may have dangerous consequences. According to confessions of certain cyclists, intravenous and subcutaneous injections are used, depending on the desired effects. It seems that doses of 50–100 IU/kg are initially used to raise the hematocrit to a limit of 50 percent and are then followed by lower doses of about 20 IU/kg.

An experimental study using intravenous doses of less than 20 IU/kg has shown that the window of detection is reduced to 12–48 hours post-injection when the criterion used is positivity of the "percentage of basic isoforms."[11] However, the sensitivity of the detection was greatly improved by the use of discriminant analysis of the EPO profiles.[7]

Whatever the sensitivity of the criteria for positivity, it is obvious that athletes have the possibility to stop an EPO treatment early enough before the beginning of a competition to escape a positive "in competition" anti-doping control. Since the lifespan of red blood cells is 4 months, the benefits of the biological effects of EPO (plasmatic half-life between 4 and 12 hours) are still felt well after all trace of the hormone has disappeared from the organism. That is why the efficiency of anti-doping control for EPO requires a strategy based on unannounced out of competition controls.

7.2 New EPOs

Since the marketing of the first recombinant EPOs, epoetin alfa (patented by Amgen in 1986) and epoetin beta (patented by Genetics Institute), several new forms of EPO have appeared. Detecting them in a urine test requires four conditions: they must be partially eliminated via the urine; they must be recognized by the antibodies used in the analysis; their isoelectric patterns must be different from that of natural urinary EPO; and the criteria for positivity must be adapted to them.

7.2.1 Biosimilar EPOs

Since 2004, the expiration of the patents protecting epoetins alfa and beta has opened the market to pharmaceutical companies interested in the production of recombinant EPO. Unlike generic drugs of chemical origin that are strictly identical to the original drug of reference, drugs that come from biotechnology present some differences from one producer to another. In some cases, differences may be observed in batches produced by the same manufacturer. These drugs cannot be qualified as "generic"; rather, they are "biosimilar."

Nonetheless, since the structures of biosimilar EPOs do not differ greatly, they are well recognized by the antibodies used for the test. As epoetins alfa and beta, they are partially eliminated in urine, and so far all of the tested isoelectric profiles have been different from that of natural urinary EPO.

The only problem for anti-doping control of biosimilars is related to the criteria for positivity. These have been originally developed to detect epoetins alfa and beta. Although the profiles of biosimilar EPOs are clearly distinguishable from that of natural urinary EPO, they may show differences from those of epoetins alfa and beta, and do not satisfy the present positivity criteria. Thus, an upgrade of these criteria is expected for the detection of biosimilar products. This concerns both the epoetins produced in the same host cell system (CHO cells) as epoetins alfa and beta and those produced in different systems such as epoetin gamma obtained from baby hamster kidney (BHK) cells or epoetin delta, produced in a human fibrosarcoma cell line. The cells used for the production of epoetin delta are not transfected with the human EPO gene that is already present in their genome. The synthesis is obtained by insertion of a promoter activating the gene encoding EPO.

This drug has given rise to great hopes of escaping a positive anti-doping control since it has been said to be identical to endogenous EPO, owing to the human origin of the host cell system used for its production. In fact, as is shown in Figure 8.8, the isoelectric pattern of this drug is different from that of the urinary endogenous EPO. However, it differs more from that of epoetin alfa than do the patterns of other biosimilar drugs, and specific positivity criteria will probably be required for its detection.

7.2.2 Modified EPOs

Besides biosimilars, modified EPOs have been developed. In comparison with the first epoetins and their biosimilars, significant changes have been introduced in their structure to increase their biological activity.

Such is the case for darbepoetin alfa (Aranesp from Amgen), a second-generation EPO. The addition of two *N*-linked carbohydrate chains means that darbepoetin alfa may have up to eight additional sialic acid residues and thus a half-life approximately three times longer than that of epoetin. This structural modification, due to a greater negative charge, seriously affects the urinary isoelectric pattern, which is clearly shifted toward more acidic pI when compared to epoetin alfa (Figure 8.2). Its detection in anti-doping control does not pose any problem since specific criteria for positivity have been developed for this special pattern. The first case reported in anti-doping control was declared during the Winter Olympic Games in Salt Lake City in 2002.[12] It is clear that since this case, athletes have rarely used darbepoetin alfa, because the longer half-life (25 hours) of this drug enhances the risks of a positive anti-doping result.

A third-generation product SEP (Synthetic Erythropoiesis Protein) has been developed by Gryphon Therapeutics and licensed by Roche but is not on sale at the present time. The originality of this form is that it is chemically synthesized and its structure is very different from that of both natural and recombinant EPOs. Essentially, this molecule is initially synthesized in the form of four independent polypeptide segments, which are then connected to each other to make a single chain of 166 amino acids. The terminal amino acid residue (arginine) is not present in natural urinary EPO, which consists of 165 amino acids. Chemical ligation of the segments is made possible by

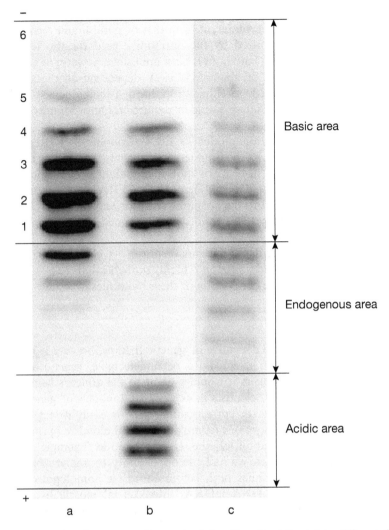

Figure 8.8 Isoelectric pattern of epoetin delta. Epoetin delta (a) is different from epoetin alfa (b) and endogenous urinary EPO (c).

substitution of glutamic acid at positions 89 and 117 by two cysteine residues. Two additional substitutions by lysine or asparagine and serine residues in positions 24 and 126 respectively allow the linking of two negatively charged polyethylylene glycol (PEG) polymer molecules. On the other hand, the important glycosylation of EPO (three sites of N-glycosylation and one site of O-glycosylation) is totally absent from SEP. This structure results in homogeneity of the synthesized SEP molecules.

The isoelectric pattern of this drug has been described as a single isoform with a pI of 5, and would thus be very easy to identify in anti-doping control. Though its structure is very different from that of natural and recombinant EPO, SEP is well recognized by the antibodies used for the test. Data concerning its metabolism have not yet been published; however, it is possible that its molecular weight of about 51–73 kD (depending on the analytical technique used) may impede its elimination through the kidneys. If it is not present in urine, a blood analysis would be required for anti-doping control of this substance.

An other third generation product, CERA (Continuous Erythropoiesis Receptor Activator) from Roche is under clinical trials. This molecule results from pegylation of Epoetin beta. Its molecular weight is about 60 kDa. It seems that unlike natural and recombinant EPO, CERA is not internalized in the cell after it has bound to the hormone receptor and thus is available for binding to other receptors. This results in a sustained erythropoietic effect and an extended half life.

As for SEP, its molecular weight may restrict its glomerular filtration. However, both for SEP and CERA, it is highly probable that the post-exercise proteinuria will favour the elimination of these molecules in urine.

7.3 Genetic doping

Presented as an inevitable derivative of genetic therapy, because it has often been predicted by certain scientists to be undetectable, genetic doping is greatly feared for the dangers it would present to the athlete's health. EPO has often been chosen by scientists in experimental models of gene therapy because the expression of the corresponding gene is easily detected by the biological effects of this hormone (stimulation of red blood cell production). Thanks to the collaboration of the Laboratoire de Thérapie Génique INSERM U649 of Nantes, we had the opportunity to analyze blood and urine samples from macaques both before and after homologous transfer of EPO complementary DNA (cDNA) into skeletal muscle by injection of adeno-associated recombinant virus (AAV).[13] The expression of the transgene was induced by doxycycline. The anti-human EPO antibodies used in the test recognize well the corresponding macaque hormone, so that it was possible to study the isoelectric patterns of the simian EPO. Induction of transgene expression in the macaque resulted in overexpression of a hormone, presenting a pattern strikingly different from that of the endogenous isoforms (Fig. 8.9).

Similar investigations were performed to study EPO gene transfer in the macaque retina. Again, the isoelectric pattern of the transgenic product was clearly different from that of the physiological EPO. Furthermore, the patterns were different depending on the cellular type transduced (retinal pigmented epithelium only or retinal pigmented epithelium and photoreceptors) and were different too from those produced by transduced skeletal

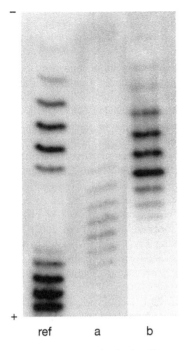

Figure 8.9 "Genetic doping." Macaque serum EPO patterns before (a) and after (b) homologous transfer of cDNA into skeletal muscle.

muscle. Skeletal muscle, being easily accessible, ought to constitute the target tissue of choice for genetic doping. Even though other systems for gene transfer must be foreseen, our observations open optimistic perspectives for detecting genetic doping.[14]

At the present time, direct detection of a banned substance is required to prove a doping offence. Detection of EPO doping has been made possible by the method described in this chapter. It may be possible to apply the same principle to the detection of other protein hormones.

8 References

1 Parisotto R, Gore CJ, Emslie KR, Ashenden MJ, Brugnara C, Howe C, Martin DT, Trout GJ, Hahn AG. A novel method utilising markers of altered erythropoiesis for the detection of recombinant human erythropoietin abuse in athletes. *Haematologica*. 2000; 85(6): 564–72.
2 Lasne F, Martin L, Crepin N, de Ceaurriz J. Detection of isoelectric profiles of erythropoietin in urine: differentiation of natural and administered recombinant hormones. *Analytical Biochemistry*. 2002; 311(2): 119–26.
3 Narhi LO, Arakawa T, Aoki KH, Elmore R, Rohde MF, Boone T, Strickland TW.

The effect of carbohydrate on the structure and stability of erythropoietin. *Journal of Biological Chemistry*. 1999; 266(34): 23022–6.

4 Lasne F. Double-blotting: a solution to the problem of non-specific binding of secondary antibodies in immunoblotting procedures. *Journal of Immunological Methods*. 2001; 253(1–2): 125–31.

5 Lasne F. Double-blotting: a solution to the problem of nonspecific binding of secondary antibodies in immunoblotting procedures *(protocol)*. *Journal of Immunological Methods*. 2003; 276(1–2): 223–6.

6 Bajla I, Holländer I, Minichmayr M, Gmeiner G, Reichel C. GASepo – a software solution for quantitative analysis of digital images in Epo doping control. *Computer Methods and Programs in Biomedicine*. 2005; 80(3): 246–70.

7 Lasne F, Thioulouse J, Martin L, de Ceaurriz J. Detection of recombinant human erythropoietin in urine for doping analysis: interpretation of isoelectric profiles by discriminant analysis. *Electrophoresis*. 2007; 28(12): 1875–81.

8 Lasne F, Martin L, de Ceaurriz J. Active urine and detection of recombinant erythropoietin. In: Schänzer W, Geyer H, Gotzmann A, Mareck U, eds. *Recent advances in doping analysis (13)*. Cologne: Sport und Buch Strauβ, 2005; 297–304.

9 Tam RC, Coleman SL, Tiplady RJ, Storring PL, Cotes PM. Comparisons of human, rat and mouse erythropoietins by isoelectric focusing: differences between serum and urinary erythropoietins. *British Journal of Haematology*. 1991; 79(3): 504–11.

10 Lasne F, Martin L, Martin JA, de Ceaurriz J. Isoelectric profiles of human erythropoietin are different in serum and urine. *International Journal of Biological Macromolecules*. 2007; 41(3): 354–7.

11 Ashenden M, Varlet-Marie E, Lasne F, Audran M. The effects of microdose recombinant human erythropoietin regimens in athletes. *Haematologica*. 2006; 91(8): 1143–4.

12 Catlin DH, Breidbach A, Elliott S, Glaspy J. Comparison of the isoelectric focusing patterns of darbepoetin alfa, recombinant human erythropoietin, and endogenous erythropoietin from human urine. *Clinical Chemistry*. 2002; 48(11): 2057–9.

13 Lasne F, Martin L, de Ceaurriz J, Larcher T, Moullier P, Chenuaud P. Genetic "doping" with erythropoietin cDNA in primate muscle is detectable. *Molecular Therapy*. 2004; 10(3): 409–10.

14 Stieger K, Le Meur G, Lasne F, Weber M, Deschamps JY, Nivard D, Mendes-Madeira A, Provost N, Martin L, Moullier P, Rolling F. Long-term doxycycline-regulated transgene expression in the retina of nonhuman primates following subretinal injection of recombinant AAV vectors. *Molecular Therapy*. 2006; 13(5): 967–75.

9 Erythrocyte volume expansion and human performance

Michael N Sawka, Stephen R Muza and Andrew J Young

1 Introduction

Erythrocyte volume expansion can be a powerful ergogenic aid which acts through multiple physiological mechanisms. Athletes have employed a variety of procedures to induce erythrocyte volume expansion to improve competitive performance. Some expansion procedures are "natural" while others are "artificial" and deemed to be unethical, and unfair to competition – and possibly to pose serious health risks.[1] The purposes of this chapter are: (1) to provide information on "normal" erythrocyte volumes in healthy adults; (2) to describe the impact of several "natural" (physical training and environmental exposure) and "artificial" (erythrocyte infusion and erythropoietin administration) methods of expanding erythrocyte volume; (3) to describe the relationship between erythrocyte volume expansion and exercise performance; and (4) to briefly review several detection approaches employed to detect "artificial" erythrocyte volume expansion, or blood doping.

2 "Normal" blood and erythrocyte volume

Blood volume represents the sum of erythrocyte volume and plasma volume. Figure 9.1 demonstrates the linear relationships between blood volume, erythrocyte volume and plasma volume relative to lean body mass (LBM).[2] These data are for healthy, active young men, and vascular volumes were measured by radioisotope labeling methodologies. Since the vascular volumes are closely related to a person's body size, normative values are generally expressed per unit body mass ($ml \cdot kg^{-1}$) or per unit lean body mass ($ml \cdot kg^{-1} \cdot LBM^{-1}$). For this active and healthy population, the mean erythrocyte volume was ~26 $ml \cdot kg^{-1}$ of body mass or ~31 $ml \cdot kg^{-1} \cdot LBM^{-1}$, the mean plasma volume was ~43 $ml \cdot kg^{-1}$ body mass or 52 $ml \cdot kg^{-1} \cdot LBW^{-1}$, and mean blood volume ~69 $ml \cdot kg^{-1}$ of body mass or 82 $ml \cdot kg^{-1} \cdot LBW^{-1}$.

In adult populations, erythrocyte volume, plasma volume and blood volume values range from 24 to 35 $ml \cdot kg^{-1}$, 38 to 49 $ml \cdot kg^{-1}$ and 62 to 84 $ml \cdot kg^{-1}$ of body weight, respectively. Women are at the lower end of this range for both erythrocyte volume and plasma volume. Figure 9.2 presents the frequency

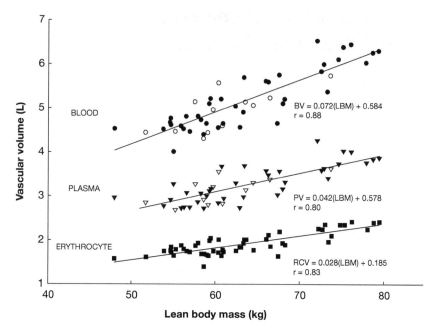

Figure 9.1 Individual data for the relationships of erythrocyte, plasma and blood
volume with lean body mass in healthy and physically fit athletes.

Source: reference 2.

distribution of the mean erythrocyte volume values from 40 studies reported in
the literature.[3] Note that although considerable overlap occurs between the
methodologies, studies employing carbon monoxide methodologies generally
yield higher values than studies employing radioactive isotopes to measure
erythrocyte volume. Therefore, some variability in the literature for erythrocyte
volume is most likely due to methodological differences, but radioactive isotope
dilution methodologies provide the reference standard.[4]

Erythrocyte volume and plasma volume measurements are technically
difficult and expensive, so simple clinical indices (e.g. venous hematocrit) are
often used to evaluate erythrocyte volume indirectly. Hematocrit is the ratio
of packed cells (mostly erythrocytes) to plasma, so it represents the proportion of blood volume that is occupied by erythrocytes. The overall hematocrit
is calculated as the ratio of measured erythrocyte volume divided by the
measured sum of erythrocyte and plasma volume. Peripheral vessel hematocrit values differ depending upon the blood collection site, because there is a
greater concentration of erythrocytes towards the blood vessel center as compared with the axis, so there is "plasma skimming" or flow of blood that is
erythrocyte poor in the smaller branching vessels. Therefore, the smaller vessels provide blood with a lower hematocrit. Venous hematocrit values are

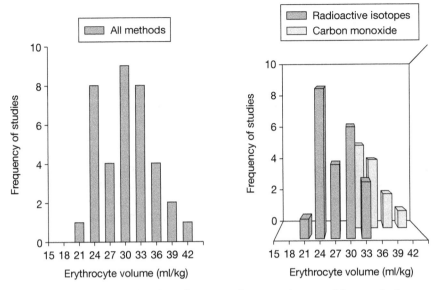

Figure 9.2 Frequency distribution of mean erythrocyte volume per kilogram body mass from 40 studies: overall distribution (left) and influence of methodology (right).

Source: reference 3.

~12 percent lower than the overall hematocrit, and this relationship is not altered by physical fitness.[2]

Since hematocrit is a ratio, it can be altered by changes in either plasma volume or erythrocyte volume, so an increased hematocrit could reflect a plasma volume reduction rather than any change in erythrocyte volume. Plasma volume is labile and is altered by hydration status, posture, prior activity and diet;[5] in contrast, erythrocyte volume is constant and naturally changes slowly over many weeks.[6] With reasonable controls for posture and hydration effects on plasma volume, the hematocrit values are relatively stable and provide reliable information on the erythrocyte volume size. Venous hematocrits are normally ~45 ± 7 (38–52 percent or points) for healthy males and ~42 ± 5 (37–47 percent or points) for healthy women, but slightly (~3–5 points) lower in physically trained and heat-acclimatized athletes because they have expanded plasma volumes.

3 Endurance training and environmental acclimatization

3.1 Endurance training

Early cross-sectional comparisons between endurance-trained and sedentary subjects suggest that blood volume is higher in trained individuals than in untrained individuals. Most longitudinal investigations report that both plasma volume and erythrocyte volume increase with endurance training; however, measurements in different studies were made at different durations, making it difficult to understand the time-frame for changes. Figure 9.3 provides results from an analysis of 18 different longitudinal studies in which all three vascular volumes were measured.[6] These results provide the average response of the three vascular volumes over time. Blood volume changes over time with exercise training demonstrate that the relative percentage change in plasma volume can increase within 24 hours following exercise and reach ~10 percent above pre-training after 1 to 4 days. In the early stage (the initial two weeks of training), nearly all blood volume expansion can be accounted for by plasma volume expansion. After ~2–3 weeks of exercise training, erythrocyte volume expansion is observed and continues to increase, until all vascular volumes reach ~8–10 percent above the pre-training baseline. As a result of this new equilibrium between plasma and erythrocyte volumes, hematocrit is most likely reestablished at its pre-training value, while blood volume is larger.

3.2 Heat acclimatization

Heat acclimatization is induced by repeated exercise-heat exposure that is sufficiently stressful to elevate both core and skin temperatures and elicit profuse sweating.[7] Erythrocyte volume does not appear to be altered by heat acclimation or season. In contrast, plasma volume is usually expanded after heat acclimation. Resting plasma volume expanded by ~5 percent (with a larger

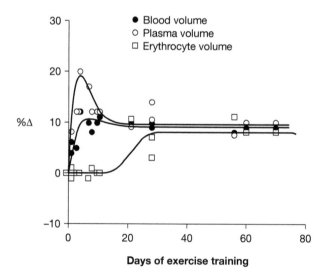

Figure 9.3 Estimated time course of relative (percentage) changes in blood volume, plasma volume and erythrocyte volume with exercise training. Data are a compilation of 18 studies.[6]

expansion during the initial week of acclimatization) in the hottest months and contracted by ~3 percent in the coldest months for people who were active outdoors.[3] As a result of plasma volume expansion associated with heat acclimatization, an athlete's hematocrit values will be lowered by several points.

3.3 Altitude acclimatization

Blood volume adjustments during altitude acclimatization have two phases.[6] In the early phase, plasma volume decreases, beginning within hours after arrival at high altitude, while erythrocyte volume remains stable. The magnitude of the plasma volume reduction is proportional to the elevation of exposure (Figure 9.4). Therefore, with altitude exposure a person's hematocrit increases while their blood volume decreases, which gives the false impression of a rapid erythrocyte volume expansion. This early phase of blood volume adjustment persists for at least three to four weeks. If altitude exposure continues for beyond a few weeks, then erythrocyte volume slowly expands. Development of the second phase may be accelerated in some lowlanders who undergo an intense aerobic training program while at altitude.[8] Erythrocyte volume expansion with prolonged high-altitude exposure is most likely fairly modest and occurs slowly over many weeks and months.[6,8]

3.4 Live at high altitude and train at lower altitudes

Athletes living (~20 h/d) at moderately high altitude (~2400 m) for three to four weeks and training hard at a lower elevation (1250 m) often exhibit a modest erythrocyte volume expansion (~35 ml/week), while subjects training similarly at sea level will exhibit no change.[8,9] Figure 9.5 shows the effects of living at moderate altitude while training at low altitude (sea level) on erythrocyte volume (red cell mass) expansion during field (Mountain House) and

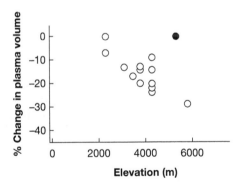

Figure 9.4 Plasma volume (percentage change) reduction associated with lowlanders acclimatizing to different altitudes. Data are a compilation of 15 studies.[6]

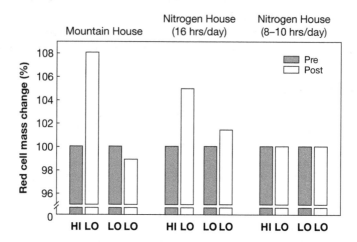

Figure 9.5 Effects of living at high altitude and training at low altitude on erythrocyte volume (red cell mass) expansion during field (Mountain House) and laboratory-simulated altitude (Nitrogen House) studies. With permission from Levine and Stray-Gundersen.[8]

simulated-altitude laboratory (Nitrogen House) studies.[8] The erythrocyte expansion associated with "living high and training low" is associated with improved aerobic exercise performance. It is of note that ~50 percent of competitive athletes studied have been identified as "nonresponders" who do not expand their erythrocyte volume, and those same subjects do not improve their aerobic exercise performance.[8,9] The mechanisms underlying the large variability in erythrocyte and performance responsiveness have not been discerned.

4 Blood doping and human performance

4.1 Blood doping

Erythrocyte volume can be artificially increased either by administering erythropoietin (EPO) and related pharmacological products or by infusing erythrocytes. In addition, future blood dopers may use oxygen-carrying blood substitutes. EPO is naturally produced, primarily in the kidneys, and stimulates erythrocyte production in bone marrow. Administering recombinant erythropoietin (rhEPO) and analogues (e.g. darbepoetin) will stimulate erythrocyte production and slowly expand erythrocyte volume. The maximal rate of erythrocyte expansion from EPO stimulation is ~50 ml/wk, and expansion will be sustained if treatment continues.[10] EPO administration most likely induces some plasma volume reduction, so interpreting hematocrit changes alone can overestimate the magnitude of erythrocyte volume expansion.[10]

Autologous erythrocytes infusion (cells produced by oneself) or homologous erythrocyte infusion (cells produced by another person) will rapidly expand erythrocyte volume, but the elevated levels will be sustained only for a few weeks. For autologous or homologous infusions, blood units are removed by phlebotomy; erythrocytes are harvested, stored and later reinfused. Blood storage and handling techniques are important as they influence erythrocyte function and survival rate, which contributes to inter-study dose–response variability. Glycerol freezing techniques allow prolonged erythrocyte storage without degradation; while refrigeration is used for short-term storage as erythrocytes will progressively degrade. Erythrocyte infusions can induce a compensatory plasma volume reduction or plasma volume expansion that is probably related to the availability of extravascular protein.[11] Therefore, hematocrit changes alone do not provide quantitative insight into the magnitude of erythrocyte volume expansion after erythrocyte infusion.

4.2 Human performance

Erythrocyte volume expansion will increase an athlete's maximal aerobic power (or maximal oxygen uptake).[12,13] A high maximal aerobic power is important in order to succeed in athletic events requiring sustained activity at high metabolic rates, and therefore erythrocyte infusion can improve athletic performance in those types of activities. Figure 9.6 presents individual data for maximal

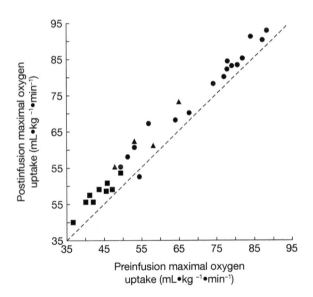

Figure 9.6 Individual data for maximal aerobic power values measured before and after erythrocyte infusion (autologous infusion of product from 2 blood units).

Source: reference 14.

aerobic power values measured before and after erythrocyte infusion (autologous infusion) of product from 2 blood units.[14] Note that 29 of 30 subjects demonstrated an increased maximal aerobic power after erythrocyte infusion, and the improvement was observed over a broad range of fitness levels. Infusing the erythrocyte product of 2 blood units will increase maximal aerobic power by ~4–11 percent, and infusing the erythrocyte product of 3–5 blood units will produce additional increases in maximal aerobic power.[1] Erythrocyte infusion and EPO administration provide similar improvements in maximal aerobic power for a given increase of hemoglobin.[15] The relationship between the magnitude of increase in hemoglobin/hematocrit, and the corresponding magnitude of increase in maximal aerobic power after blood doping, are strong with group mean analyses, but are often weak for individual subject analyses.

Aerobic performance improvements from erythrocyte volume expansion are primarily mediated by increased oxygen-carrying capacity of the blood; thus, a lower cardiac output is needed to deliver a given amount of oxygen to the active skeletal muscles. During submaximal (steady-state) exercise, the muscle oxygen delivery requirements will be achieved by using less cardiac reserve and endurance will thereby be improved. In addition, erythrocyte volume expansion will improve acid-base buffering capabilities as well as improve heat loss responses which mediate reduced heat storage during exercise-heat stress and an improved ability to tolerate dehydration.[11]

5 Detection of blood doping

The testing of athletes for artificial erythrocyte volume expansion or "blood doping" includes a variety of blood and perhaps urine tests. These tests will need to be conducted on multiple occasions during each year and to include pre-event values, to account for differences in seasons (differences in heat acclimatization status) and training practices.

Blood doping can be evaluated by screening for specific hematological parameters (e.g. hemoglobin, hematocrit, reticulocyte count and indices, soluble transferring receptor) which are sensitive to blood doping and then following these and other pertinent parameters over many months or years. This will enable the development of an individual "hematological passport" profile with upper thresholds that can be used to identify trends associated with blood doping.[16] In addition, mathematical models employing many of these hematological parameters appear to have great potential to identify athletes who are blood doping.[17] An alternative approach to detect blood doping is to screen for recombinant erythropoietin and analogues in the blood or urine.[18–21] However, this approach is highly dependent upon the timing of the sample collection in relation to the administration and subsequent pharmacokinetics.[22] Future blood doping tests will most likely include molecular biology approaches, including transcriptional profiling.[23]

6 Summary

Erythrocyte volume expansion is a powerful ergogenic aid that can be induced by "natural" and "artificial" procedures. Erythrocyte volume measurements are technically difficult and expensive to carry out, so hematocrit is often used to evaluate erythrocyte volume indirectly; however, interpretation of repeated hematocrit measures can be confounded by plasma volume changes. Erythrocyte volume is naturally increased slowly by endurance (aerobic) training and high-altitude exposure; whereas heat stress and cold stress exposure will rapidly alter plasma volume without changing erythrocyte volume. Erythrocyte volume can be artificially increased slowly by administering erythropoietin (EPO) and related pharmacological products or be rapidly increased by infusing erythrocytes. Almost every subject who increases their erythrocyte volume will increase their aerobic exercise performance capability, and this ergogenic advantage is some-what proportionate to the magnitude of erythrocyte volume expansion. A variety of blood and urine tests are becoming more effective in identifying athletes who employ "artificial" erythrocyte volume expansion or "blood doping."

DISCLAIMER: The views expressed in this chapter are those of the authors and do not reflect the official policy of the Department of the Army, Department of Defense or the US Government.

7 References

1 Sawka MN, Joyner MJ, Robertson RJ, Spriet LL, Young AJ. The use of blood doping as an ergogenic aid: ACSM position stand. *Medicine and Science in Sports and Exercise*. 1996; 28(6): i–viii.
2 Sawka MN, Young AJ, Pandolf KB, Dennis RC, Valeri CR. Erythrocyte, plasma and blood volume of healthy young men. *Medicine and Science in Sports and Exercise*. 1992; 24: 447–53.
3 Sawka, MN, Coyle EF. Influence of body water and blood volume on thermoregulation and exercise-heat performance. In: Holloszy JO, ed. *Exercise and Sport Sciences Reviews*. Baltimore: Williams & Wilkins, 1999; 27: 167–218.
4 International Committee for Standardization in Hematology. Recommended methods for measurement of red-cell and plasma volume. (1980) *Journal of Nuclear Medicine*. 1980; 21: 793–800.
5 Mack GW. The body fluid and hemopoietic systems. In Tipton CM, Sawka MN, Tate CA, Terjung RL, eds. *ACSM's Advanced Exercise Physiology*. Baltimore: Lippincott Williams & Wilkins, 2006; 501–31.
6 Sawka MN, Convertino VA, Eichner ER, Schnieder SM, Young AJ. Blood volume: Importance and adaptations to exercise training, environmental stresses and trauma/sickness. *Medicine and Science in Sports and Exercise*. 2000; 32: 332–48.
7 Sawka MN, Young AJ. Physiological systems and their responses to conditions of heat and cold. In: Tipton CM, Sawka MN, Tate CA, Terjung RL, eds. *ACSM's Advanced Exercise Physiology*. Baltimore: Lippincott Williams & Wilkins, 2006; 535–63.

8 Levine BD, Stray-Gundersen J. Dose response of altitude training: How much altitude is enough? In: Roach RC, Wagner PD, Hackett PH, eds. *Advances in Experimental Medicine and Biology: Hypoxia and exercise.* New York: Springer Science, 2006; 233–47.

9 Mazzeo RS, Fulco CS. Physiological systems and their responses to conditions of hypoxia. In: Tipton CM, Sawka MN, Tate CA, Terjung RL, eds. *ACSM Advanced Exercise Physiology.* 2006; 564–80.

10 Berglund B, Eklund B. Effects of recombinant erythropoietin treatment on blood pressure and some hematological parameters in healthy men. *Journal of Internal Medicine.* 1991; 229: 125–30.

11 Sawka MN, Young AJ. (1989) Acute polycythemia and human performance during exercise and exposure to extreme environments. In: Holloszy JO, ed. *Exercise and Sport Sciences Reviews.* Baltimore: Williams & Wilkins, 17: 265–93.

12 Buick FJ, Gledhill N, Froese AB, Spriet L, Meyers EC. Effect of induced erythro-cythemia on aerobic work capacity. *Journal of Applied Physiology.* 1980; 48: 636–42.

13 Celsing F, Svedenhag J, Pihlstedt P, Ekblom B. (1987) Effects of anemia and stepwise-induced polycythaemia on maximal aerobic power in individuals with high and low haemoglobin concentrations. *Acta Physiologica Scandinavica.* 1987; 129: 47–57.

14 Sawka MN, Young AJ, Muza SR, Gonzalez RR, Pandolf KB. Erythrocyte reinfu-sion and maximal aerobic power: An examination of modifying factors. *Journal of the American Medical Association.* 1987; 257: 1496–9.

15 Ekblom B, Berglund B. Effect of erythropoietin administration on maximal aerobic power. *Scandinavian Journal of Medicine and Science in Sports.* 1991; 1: 88–93.

16 Malcovati L, Cazzola M. Hematologic passport for athletes competing in endurance sports: a feasibility study. *Haematologica.* 2003; 88: 570–81.

17 Gore CJ, Parisotto R, Ashenden MJ, Stray-Gunderson J, Hopkins W, Emslie KR, Howe C, Trout GJ, Kazlauskas R, Hahn AG. (2003) Second generation blood tests to detect erythropoietin abuse by athletes. *Haematologica.* 2003; 88: 333–44.

18 Parisotto R, Wu M, Ashenden MJ, Emslie KR, Gore C, Howe C, Kazlauskas R, Sharpe K, Trout GJ, Xie M, Hahn AG. Detection of recombinant human erythro-poietin abuse in athletes utilizing markers of altered erythropoiesis. *Haematologica.* 2001; 86: 128–37.

19 Catlin DH, Breidbach A, Elliott S, Gaspy J. Comparison of the isoelectric focusing patterns of darbepoetin alfa, recombinant human erythropoietin, and endogenous erythropoietin from human urine. *Clinical Chemistry.* 2002; 48: 2057–9.

20 Lasne F, de Ceaurriz J. Recombinant erythropoietin in urine. *Nature.* 2000; 405: 635–7.

21 Morkeberg JS, Lundby C, Nissen-Lie G, Nielsen TK, Hemmersbach P, Damsgaard R. Detection of darbepoetin alfa misuse in urine and blood. *Medicine and Science in Sports and Exercise.* 2007; 39: 1742–7.

22 Ramakrishnan R, Cheung WK, Wacholtz MC, Minton N, Jusko WJ. Pharmacokinetic and pharmacodynamic modeling of recombinant human erythropoietin after single and multiple doses in healthy volunteers. *Journal of Clinical Pharmacology.* 2004; 44: 991–1002.

23 Fedoruk MN, Rupert JL. Development of a prototype blood-based test for exoge-nous erythropoietin activity based on transcriptional profiling. Presented at IAAF World Anti-Doping Symposium, Lausanne, 2006.

10 Growth Hormone, Secretogogues and related issues

Peter Sönksen and Richard Holt

1 Introduction

Growth hormone (GH) is a naturally occurring endogenous peptide hormone produced by the pituitary gland. It has strong anabolic properties regulating body composition and is widely believed to be a major drug of abuse in sport. Its use is banned by the International Olympic Committee (IOC) and it appears on the World Anti-Doping Agency (WADA) list of prohibited substances.

The detection of exogenously administered GH is challenging, as it is almost identical to the GH produced naturally by the pituitary gland. Furthermore, the pulsatile secretion of GH leads to wide variations in circulating GH concentrations, not least in the post-competition setting where exercise acts as a potent stimulus for GH secretion.

Despite these difficulties, a test with good sensitivity and specificity has been developed and should ensure that athletes doping with GH are no longer able to use the substance with impunity. This chapter will examine the history of doping with GH and the projects to catch the GH cheats.

2 History

Growth hormone was the name given to an extract of human pituitary glands that was purified by Li *et al.* in 1945[1] and shown to promote growth in hypopituitary animals. This extract was soon used to treat children with hypopituitarism, dramatically restoring growth.[2] Observations were made regarding the beneficial effects in adults as early as 1962:

> Replacement therapy with thyroid, adrenocortical hormone and estrogen in females or androgens in males is usually satisfactory treatment for adult hypopituitarism. One patient, a thirty-five year old teacher, treated in this way for eight years, was treated in addition with human growth hormone, 3 mg three times a week. After two months of GH she noted increased vigor, ambition and sense of well-being. Observations in more cases will be needed to indicate whether the favorable effect was more than coincidental.[3]

It was not until 20 years later, however, that it was first recommended in the underground market as a performance-enhancing drug,[4] and not until 25 years later that its role in regulating body composition in human adults in such a way that it might be regarded as a new anabolic agent was appreciated by the medical profession.[5,6] Thus, as is often the case in the history of sport, the athletes got there before the scientists!

Growth hormone extracted from human pituitary glands was the only source of the hormone until 1987, when the first recombinant version (methionyl human GH) became available. The recognition that pituitary-derived GH was a source for the prion-induced Creutzfeldt-Jakob disease led to its withdrawal from the marketplace in 1985,[7] although supplies of pituitary-derived GH continue to be available on the black market to this day.

3 Growth hormone physiology

GH is secreted from the anterior pituitary in a pulsatile manner under the control of the hypothalamic hormones GH-releasing hormone (GHRH), somatostatin and ghrelin. GH is the most abundant pituitary hormone, and the human pituitary contains 5–10 mg. GH exists as multiple isoforms: 75 percent of circulating GH is in the form of a 22-kD polypeptide while 5–10 percent is in the 20-kD isoform, as a result of mRNA splicing. Several posttranslational modifications such as acylation also occur.

3.1 Regulation of GH secretion

GHRH and ghrelin stimulate the synthesis and release of GH, while somato-statin is inhibitory in action. Although ghrelin is secreted by the hypothalamus, its major source is the stomach. It is thought to be one mechanism that controls the GH response to eating, but also has an important role in the control of eating behavior.

There are a number of physiological conditions that stimulate and inhibit GH release, the most important of which are exercise and sleep (Table 10.1). The highest GH peaks occur at night within the first hour of sleep (slow-wave sleep).[8] The wide physiological variation in GH concentrations was a major challenge in developing a test for GH abuse.

3.2 Effects of growth hormone deficiency and replacement

The physiological effects of GH in adults are best examined by considering the condition of GH deficiency and the effects of GH replacement. Until 1989, when the first studies on GH replacement in adults were published, it was believed that gonadal steroids were the most important hormones regulating body composition. It is now appreciated that GH also plays a piv-otal role, because in the absence of GH, lean tissue is lost and fat accumulates.

Table 10.1 Regulation of endogenous GH secretion by the pituitary

Stimulation	Inhibition
GH-releasing hormone	Somatostatin
Ghrelin	
Puberty	Ageing
Sleep	Obesity
Exercise	
Hypoglycaemia	Hyperglycaemia
Reduced FFA	Increased free fatty acids (FFA)
Increased amino acids	
Oestrogens	GH
Androgens	Raised IGF-I
	Progesterone
	Glucocorticoids
α-Adrenergic agonists	β-Adrenergic agonists
Serotonin	Serotonin antagonists
Dopamine agonists	Dopamine antagonists

Waist to hip ratio increases as visceral fat increases. While in children, the most obvious sign of GH deficiency is poor linear growth, the effects in adults are broader, reflecting the major role of GH in multiple systems.

Until the advent of recombinant technology, GH was scarce and in most countries carefully "rationed" for use only in children with GH deficiency. The availability of potentially unlimited amounts of recombinant human growth hormone (rhGH) in the late 1980s led to an upsurge in interest by the pharmaceutical industry as it saw the potential for a wider and more lucrative market. Two seminal papers published in 1989[5,6] confirmed beyond any doubt the importance of GH in adults as well as in children. These independent studies, undertaken in Denmark and the United Kingdom, used double-blind placebo-controlled trials in adults with hypopituitarism given appropriate replacement therapy with everything apart from GH. Jorgensen and colleagues used a "crossover" design while Salomon *et al.* used a "parallel group" design. Both used six months of treatment with active drug or placebo, and the findings were remarkably congruous, thus enhancing their impact.

Perhaps the most impressive finding was a change in body composition, with an average increase of 6 kg of lean body mass (LBM) with a concomitant loss of a similar amount of fat. This "normalised" the body composition of the GH-deficient patients. Salomon *et al.* also looked at "quality of life" using a panel of four questionnaires and found marked improvements, particularly in the area of "increased energy".[9] Many patients commented that the treatment restored them to normal living, whereas previously they "just existed."

Using CT scanning of the thighs, the increases in LBM were shown to be largely accounted for by increases in muscle bulk, and exercise studies revealed the expected enhancements in performance.[10,11] Later studies showed that exercise performance continued to improve over the first three years of GH replacement,[12] and the normalisation of body composition was effected through

Table 10.2 Effects of growth hormone in adults

Effect of GH deficiency	Effect of GH replacement
Body composition	
Increased body fat	Decreased body fat
Increased waist:hip ratio (WHR)	Decreased WHR
Increased visceral fat mass	Decreased visceral fat mass
Decreased lean body mass	Increased lean body mass
Decreased bone mineral density	Increased bone mineral density
Physical performance	
Decreased muscle mass	Increased muscle mass
Decreased muscle strength	Increased muscle strength
Decreased maximal exercise performance	Increased maximal exercise performance
Decreased maximum oxygen uptake	Increased VO_2 max, maximum power
Decreased maximum heart rate	output, maximum heart rate and anaerobic threshold
Psychological well-being	Increased energy levels
Decreased ability to cope with daily life	Increased ability to participate in
Decreased physical and mental energy	physical activities without tiring
Decreased concentration skills	Improved emotional reactions
Decreased initiative	Less social isolation
Increased social isolation	Increased perceived quality of life
Decreased self-esteem	Increased self-esteem
Decreased sex life	Decreased sleep requirement
Increased sleep requirement	
Increased level of perceived health problems	
Heart	
Increased mortality	Increased red cell mass
Increased prevalence of cardiovascular events	Increased left ventricular mass
	Increased stroke volume
Increased hypertension	Increased cardiac output and resting
Decreased left ventricular mass	heart rate
Decreased fibre shortening	Decreased diastolic blood pressure

stimulation of protein synthesis.[13] There were also favourable changes in lipid metabolism[14] and in erythropoesis[15] with resultant increase in plasma volume and red cell mass. From these placebo-controlled studies it was possible to identify the entirely new syndrome "Growth Hormone Deficiency in Adults (GHDA)," with a well-defined set of symptoms, signs and biochemical findings.[16]

These studies furthered our understanding of GH as a "partitioning agent." In both humans and animals, GH determines where and how ingested energy is stored in the body and thus regulates body composition in adults. The importance of this with regard to doping in sport became clear to sports physiologists and scientists some seven years before it appeared in the medical literature.

3.3 Mechanism of action

Growth hormone receptors seem to be present on every cell in the body. Growth hormone binds with two receptors to activate a protein kinase cascade and eventually stimulate amino acid uptake and protein synthesis,[17] while testosterone and oestradiol act through nuclear receptors and an entirely separate signalling system. Since they operate through separate and distinct pathways, it seems likely that their effects will be additive, and indeed that has been shown to be the case. The regulation of protein synthesis also involves the synergistic actions of GH and IGF-I stimulating protein synthesis, while there is a simultaneous inhibition of protein breakdown by insulin.[18] (Figure 10.1).

3.4 Effects of growth hormone excess

Studies of GH-deficient adults are important in helping us understand the normal physiological role of GH in adults as a "partitioning agent" but this does not mean that administering GH to normal adults or elite athletes will necessarily be "performance enhancing." Indeed, Nature's experiment of excess GH administration to adults – acromegaly, usually caused by excessive GH secretion from a benign pituitary tumour – is usually associated with muscle weakness rather than excessive strength. It needs to be appreciated, however,

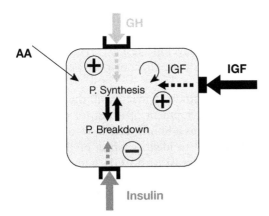

Figure 10.1 Our current understanding about the synergistic action between insulin, IGF-I and GH in regulating protein (P) synthesis. Without insulin, GH loses much (if not all) of its anabolic action. The anabolic action of both GH and IGF-I appears to be mediated through induction of amino acid (AA) transporters in the cell membrane. This is reflected *in vivo* through an increase of amino acid metabolic clearance rate. It is not yet clear how much of IGF-I's action is through locally generated IGF-I ("autocrine" and "paracrine") or through circulating IGF-I that is largely derived from the liver.

that acromegaly invariably goes unnoticed for a long time (on average 10–15 years) before a diagnosis is made. Many patients, if questioned carefully, will give a history of increased strength in the early stage (first few years) of their condition. Indeed, a medical practitioner known personally to the authors was an elite rower while an undergraduate at Oxbridge when he was in the early stages of acromegaly. He found that not only was he one of the strongest members of the team but also he was able to tolerate harder training sessions than his colleagues and recovered more quickly afterwards. Of course, this is only a clinical anecdote, but it is in keeping with recognised effects of GH and illustrates that the lack of abnormal strength in acromegalic patients at the time of diagnosis tells us nothing except that tremendous excess of GH (levels are 10- to 1000-fold higher than normal) over many years leads to muscle weakness. Indeed, early death from cardiomyopathy is not uncommon in young people with acromegaly with very high GH levels. It is well recognised in human physiology (and pharmacology) that a dose-response curve often peaks at a given optimum dose and then falls when the dose is increased further; this is probably what happens in acromegaly. Furthermore, acromegaly is often accompanied by deficiencies of other pituitary hormones, such as ACTH, with resultant hypoadrenalism that may affect physical performance.

4 Administration of growth hormone to normal people

When given in supraphysiological doses for one to four weeks to normal, fit, endurance-trained adults, GH produces effects in keeping with those expected in the light of the effects of GH seen in GHDA, apart from the fact that there was until very recently no study confirming a performance enhancing effect.[19] The GH-2000 project, whose aim was to develop a test for GH abuse, included double-blind placebo-controlled studies of the effect of rhGH administration to amateur athletes.

The first study was a one-week pilot study to identify all the GH-sensitive markers that might be useful in the development of a test for detecting GH abuse. A quantity of 0.15 IU/kg rhGH was administered daily to a small number of endurance-trained young men[20,21] to identify which of the more than 25 blood markers evaluated were most sensitive to GH administration but not to acute exercise. Ten of these markers (Figure 10.2) were further evaluated in a second, larger double-blind placebo-controlled study in which rhGH was administered to over 100 endurance-trained amateur male and female athletes from four European countries at doses of 0.1 and 0.2 IU/kg.[22,23] Although these studies were primarily designed to develop a test for GH abuse, they also provided an opportunity to examine the effects of long-term GH administration in normal young individuals.

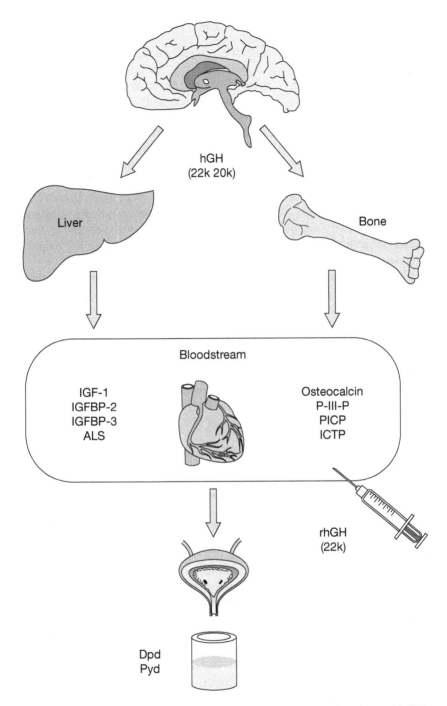

Figure 10.2 Growth hormone-sensitive markers evaluated for detecting abuse with GH. See text for meaning of abbreviations. Dpd is deoxypyridinoline crosslinks and Pyd is pyridinium crosslinks

4.1 Effects of growth hormone on metabolism

These studies of rhGH administration to endurance-trained athletes showed that GH stimulates protein metabolism both at rest and during exercise,[24] and at the same time mobilises energy from stored fat by stimulating lipolysis.[25] If growth hormone has a performance-enhancing effect, it is most likely through these linked mechanisms. Stimulation of protein synthesis leads over time to increased muscle size and strength, while by inhibiting protein oxidation during exercise and simultaneously mobilising free fatty acids (as an alternative fuel to glucose), it helps to make training and exercise an anabolic activity.[26]

Despite agreement about its extensive abuse in sport, there is controversy over growth hormone's ability to be a performance-enhancing substance.[27] Indeed, not everyone believes it has protein anabolic actions in normal humans,[28] although this opinion seems to be at variance with the balance of the modern scientific literature.

Hintz's editorial in the *British Medical Journal*[27] also doubts a potential role of GH's anabolic actions in the management of frailty in the aged, although a recent double-blind placebo-controlled trial of GH, testosterone or GH plus testosterone in 80 healthy elderly men showed GH to be a more potent anabolic agent than testosterone. GH and testosterone had an additive effect not only on body composition but also on quality of life, strength and exercise performance[29] (Figure 10.3). More recently, a well-designed and well-executed study in past abusers of anabolic steroids showed for the first time an ergogenic effect of GH in healthy athletes.[30] Although it is likely that this issue will remain controversial, it should be borne in mind that conventional randomised controlled trials have most often been underpowered to detect the small differences in performances needed by an athlete to achieve a gold medal.

5 Doping with growth hormone: history

How and where GH was first used as a doping agent is not clear, but the first publication to draw attention to it was a cyclostyled news-sheet emerging from California under the editorship of Dan Duchaine in 1982.[4] The description of the actions of GH that appeared in this article was remarkably accurate, suggesting he had access to expert medical advice. Although there were some fundamental errors, such as recommending (and advertising for sale) animal growth hormone for use in man, it gave a very accurate, albeit somewhat exaggerated, account of its protein anabolic effects, none of which had yet appeared in the conventional medico-scientific literature.

In 1988, Ben Johnson won a gold medal in the 100 metres at the Olympic Games in Seoul. He was subsequently disqualified after stanazolol was detected in his urine, and both he and his coach, Charley Francis, admitted under oath that he had taken human growth hormone in addition to anabolic steroids.

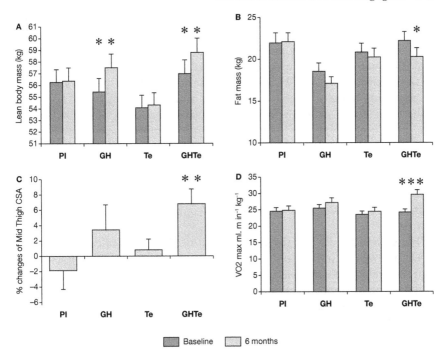

Figure 10.3 The effects of placebo, GH, testosterone (Te), and combined GH and Te on lean body mass (A), fat mass (B), percentage change from 0 to 6 months in the mid-thigh cross-sectional area (C), and VO$_2$ max (D). In A, B and D the dark shading indicates the baseline and the lighter shading the reading after 6 months. *, $P < 0.02$; **, $P < 0.01$; ***, $P < 0.001$.

Source: reference 29.

By 1991, the International Olympic Committee (IOC) realised that the issue of GH needed to be addressed, and one of the authors (PHS) received a telephone call from Professor Manfred Donike on behalf of Prince Alexander de Merode, chairman of the IOC Medical Commission, inviting him to join the IOC Medical Commission's Sub-Commission "Doping and Biochemistry in Sport" as an adviser on growth hormone. Growth hormone was discussed by the IOC for the first time at a meeting of the Medical Commission and Sub-Commission in Lillehammer a year before the 1994 Winter Games. This meeting was an illuminating introduction to the workings of the IOC and made it clear that developing a test to detect GH abuse was not going to be just a straightforward piece of scientific research. The Chairman of the Medical Commission and Sub-Commission was a layman who had absorbed a considerable amount of medical and scientific knowledge through his lifetime dedicated to building the anti-doping structure of the IOC. In this activity he had a stalwart scientific partner in Professor Manfred Donike; between them they had developed a worldwide network of top-class laboratories staffed by top-grade chemists and pharma-cologists. At this time, the IOC laboratories and scientific staff were equipped to measure mainly steroids and stimulants in urine and had limited experience in dealing with the more complex protein and glycoprotein hormones.

To establish a test for GH, the first requirement was for blood rather than urine testing. Initially the concept of blood testing was greeted with horror, as hitherto all testing had been performed on urine samples. In fact, blood testing was introduced a year later at the Lillehammer Olympic Games in 1994 (much against the wishes of the chairman of the IOC Medical Commission) under the auspices of the International Ski Federation (FIS) for the detection of "blood doping" (heterologous blood transfusions). Much to the surprise of those strongly opposed to blood testing, the whole process ran smoothly without a hitch and was indeed much less trouble than the conventional urine testing.

The second hurdle was the concept of a need for scientific research to be done to develop a suitable test. There was a general feeling within IOC circles that research on athletes was unacceptable because of the need to protect the athletes from the potential "threat" of the scientists after their body fluids. To a newcomer recruited to help solve what was judged by the IOC to be a new and important problem, this was not easy to understand, but Professor Donike (who was secretary of the Sub-Commission, but *de facto* in charge of its scientific operations) went to great lengths to explain the workings of the IOC and the challenges to be met, and to help PHS develop a strategy to over-come them. Without his support and encouragement (and later, the support of the president-to-be Jacques Rogge), no research would ever have been done with IOC involvement.

There was also a need to update the knowledge of the Medical Commission about the normal physiological role of GH as well as its potential ergogenic actions and some possible approaches to developing a suitable test. An opportunity to do so presented itself in February 1991 at a meeting of the Sub-Commission and the full Medical Commission. There was lively interest, and many questions were asked, particularly about the potential of GH in the elderly.

Although a greater understanding for the need for research was obtained at the meeting, a major issue arose because the IOC did not fund research, in par-ticular "invasive" clinical science, and it was not clear where suitable funding could be found. It was definitely not the sort of research normally funded by conventional sources of grants for medical research, such as research councils or charities, and industrial firms were not interested in funding research on an unlicensed use of their product. This presented a big problem as this was a clear example of "commissioned" research where the appropriate "commis-sioner" was not prepared to find the resources needed as they felt that this was not their role. The actual word "research" was so disliked by the IOC that it became taboo and so the code "development" was used, as this word seemed acceptable to the IOC.

Over the next three years, constant gentle pressure from the IOC Sub-Commission managed to convert Prince de Merode to the view that "development" was a necessary evil in order to get a job done. Using his influence to lobby the research arm of the European Union (EU) in Brussels (in partnership with a fellow Belgian, orthopaedic surgeon, Olympic silver medallist and IOC member and now president Jacques Rogge), Prince de Merode persuaded the EU to include in its Biomedicine and Health (BIOMED 2) 1994–8 research programme "Area 1 – Pharmaceuticals Research" a task "1.1 Phamacotoxicology" and a sub-task "1.1.8 Research in pharmaceutical aspects of illicit drug demand reduction, including doping in sports."[31]

This truly "commissioned" research initiative by the EU was an ideal opportunity to seek funding for a research project to develop a test for GH in sport, and "GH-2000" was conceived. The GH-2000 project consisted of a consortium of leading endocrinologists with expertise in GH research from four European countries (United Kingdom, Sweden, Denmark and Italy), in partnership with two pharmaceutical companies manufacturing GH (Novo Nordisk (Denmark) and Pharmacia (Sweden)), statisticians from the University of Kent (United Kingdom) and the IOC Medical Commission. The proposal was submitted in spring 1995 and approved in the fall of 1995 but at only one-third of the US$3 million budget sought. Probably as a result of some fortunate misunderstanding about the role and responsibility of the IOC with the EU and the project, the chairman of the IOC Medical Commission came to the rescue by finding a matching additional US$1 million from the IOC, and the project was born on January 1, 1996 after a three-year gestation period.[32] So, for the first time the IOC funded "invasive" scientific research.

6 The science behind the detection of GH abuse

In addition to the need for blood testing because of the unpredictable and erratic excretion of GH by the kidney, there are several aspects that make the development of a test for GH challenging. Exogenous recombinant human GH (rhGH) and endogenous GH have identical amino acid sequences, making chemical distinction impossible. In normal individuals, serum GH concentrations vary widely throughout the day. GH is secreted in a pulsatile manner and is under the influence of stress, exercise, sleep and food intake. This pattern of secretion results in serum concentrations that vary widely throughout the day and frequently overlap with measurements obtained following exogenous administration of GH.

Two main approaches have been investigated to detect GH abuse. The first, developed by the GH-2000 team, relies on measurement of GH-dependent markers, while the second, pioneered by Professor Christian Strasburger and his team in Germany, is based on the detection of different pituitary GH isoforms. They are quite different in concept but are complementary rather than competitive in nature.

6.1 GH-dependent markers

6.1.1 The GH-2000 project

The GH-2000 project ran for three years, from January 1996 to January 1999, and was aimed at delivering the methodology for a suitable test to the IOC in time for implementation at the 2000 Olympic Games in Sydney, Australia. It was based on a model identifying physiological substances or combinations of substances that are sensitive to the effects of GH but not exercise, whose presence in the bloodstream or urine at concentrations greater than those possible under "normal physiological circumstances" would be pathognemonic for GH abuse.

It had four components:

1   A cross-sectional study with collection of blood samples taken within two hours of competition from a large population of elite athletes at national or international events to establish reference ranges of the selected "markers" of GH action;
2   A pilot "Wash-out Study" where blood samples were collected during and after one week's rhGH administration to recreational male athletes to identify the most suitable "markers" of GH action;
3   A GH administration study involving self-administered rhGH (at two doses) or placebo for one month to a large group of recreational athletes under strict double-blind placebo-controlled conditions to allow evalua-tion of the potential markers for their ability to discriminate active drug from placebo and to evaluate the "window of opportunity" when the test remained positive after rhGH was stopped;
4   An injury study to investigate any potential confounding effects produced by injury or other events.

As a result of the "Wash-out study," the markers judged most suitable came either from the IGF-I axis or from bone and collagen metabolism (Figure 10.2). An ideal marker or combination of markers would have a well-defined refer-ence range with little diurnal or day-to-day variation, would rise several-fold in response to GH administration and would remain altered after GH had been discontinued. The marker should be largely unaffected by other external regu-lators of GH secretion such as exercise or injury and should be validated across populations.[33]

In the GH-2000 double-blind study, there were predictable effects of GH increasing IGF-I and its major binding proteins IGFBP-3 and ALS (acid-labile subunit), but, somewhat surprisingly, we did not see the anticipated fall in IGFBP-2 seen in a previous study.[34]

The changes in markers derived from bone and collagen metabolism were impressive and to a certain degree unexpected. Procollagen Type 3 N-terminal peptide (P-III-P) is a marker of Type 3 collagen formation, mainly in soft tissues. The C-terminal propeptide of Type 1 collagen (PICP) is involved in the early scaffold of collagen formation with bone remodelling and callus formation. The C-terminal cross-linked telopeptide of Type 1 collagen (ICTP) is a marker of bone resorption. Osteocalcin and bone alkaline phosphatase are both markers of bone mineralisation. These markers rose in a dose-dependent manner after GH administration, but the rates of rise and fall after stopping GH varied considerably between them (see Table 10.3).[21]

Following analysis of the results of these studies, the GH-2000 project proposed a test based on insulin-like growth factor I (IGF-I) and Type 3 pro-collagen (P-III-P). IGF-I and P-III-P are ideal candidate markers because they exhibit little diurnal or day-to-day variation and are largely unaffected by exercise or gender. In the GH-2000 GH administration studies, IGF-I and P-III-P rose more than threefold while in contrast rose by only 20 percent and 10.2 percent respectively following exhaustive exercise.

There was a careful evaluation of the 12 potential markers of GH action measured during the double-blind study, and although most of them had discriminatory power, ultimately IGF-I and P-III-P were chosen as the two markers that gave the best discrimination between those taking GH and those taking placebo. Although discrimination was the prime reason for the selection, it is important that these proteins are produced by different tissues, thereby reducing the number of pathological conditions that could lead to an elevation in both markers and potential false positives.

As IGF-I and P-III-P occur physiologically, proof of GH abuse must rely on detecting levels convincingly in excess of those found in an established reference range. The GH-2000 studied over 800 elite athletes in the immediate post-competition setting and derived gender-specific reference ranges.[35] Although there is little effect of sporting discipline and body composition, there is an age-related decline in both IGF-I and P-III-P which is consistent with the known fall in endogenous GH secretion with age.

Following GH administration, the marked increase in IGF-I and P-III-P leads to clear separation between those taking GH and those taking placebo. Although a single marker could be used, by combining markers in conjunction with gender-specific equations – "discriminant functions" – the sensitivity and specificity of the ability to detect GH abuse can be improved compared with

Table 10.3 Disappearance half-lives of markers of GH

Marker	Disappearance half-life (h)
Osteocalcin	770
PICP	433
P-III-P	693
ICTP	248
IGF-I	89.5
IGFBP-3	179
ALS	119

Source: Adapted from reference 35.

single-marker analysis. Thus, the basis of the proposed test was the measurement of two substances, insulin-like growth factor I (IGF-I) and procollagen Type 3 N-terminal peptide (P-III-P), and their inclusion in a formula, thereby calculating a score.

The procedure used to generate the discriminant functions involves splitting the available data into two: a smaller "training" set that is used to calculate the discriminant function, and a larger "confirmatory" set that is then used to validate the sensitivity and specificity of the discriminant function. The confirmatory set is required to ensure that the model is applicable to the general population and not just the "training" set, but the method has the limitation that it is to an extent "self-fulfilling," and validation on a completely independent dataset is really needed to confirm its reliability.

It was shown through statistical analysis that optimum discrimination between active GH and placebo groups was obtained using just two of the 12 substances examined. The addition of more markers did not enhance that statistical power. Standard medical practice accepts "normal" values as being within two standard deviations of the mean, but by definition 5 percent of the population lie outside the "normal range." This would create an unacceptably high false positive rate if applied to athletes. The specificity to be used has not been determined by the anti-doping authorities, but after a workshop with a prominent IOC lawyer, GH-2000 concluded that false positive rates of 1 in 10,000 would be acceptable.

Using IGF-I and P-III-P it was possible on day 21 of treatment to detect 23 of the 28 men on rhGH including those on the lower dose used, which was judged to be at the lower level of dosage expected to be encountered in GH abuse (Table 10.4). The ability to detect those taking GH was less easy in women than men and greatest while the subject was still taking GH but continued after discontinuing treatment for as long as 14 days, albeit at a reduced sensitivity.[36]

The lower sensitivity in women probably occurs because women are more resistant to the actions of GH. This potential disadvantage may be offset because women may need to receive higher doses to obtain a performance-enhancing benefit, and anecdotal evidence suggests that the doses used by athletes may be up to ten times higher than those used by the GH-2000 study.

The project was completed on time and within budget, and GH-2000 reported its results in confidence to the EU and IOC on 20 January, 1999.[37] It showed not only that a test was possible but exactly how it should be done. The test was relatively straightforward in scientific terms and exhibited very good sensitivity at a very high specificity and with a window of opportunity that could last as long as 14 days after the last injection of GH. In response, the IOC organised a workshop in Rome in March 1999 with invited outside experts from around the world to review critically and quality-assure the results.

The conclusion of this workshop was strong support for the results, with one prominent workshop member (a lawyer from the Court of Arbitration for

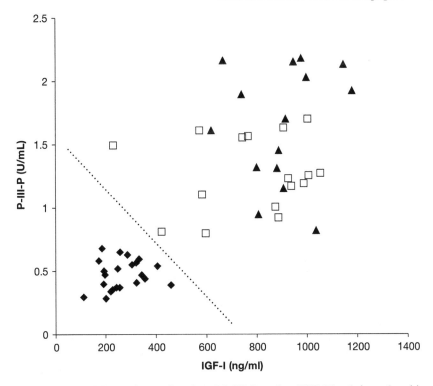

Figure 10.4 Individual data-point plot of P-III-P against IGF-I levels in male subjects after three weeks' treatment with low-dose (□) or high-dose (▲) GH or placebo (◆).

Table 10.4 Effects of specificity on the sensitivity of the marker method in men and women

Cut-off value	Approximate specificity of test	Success rate according to day after commencing GH					
		Day 21 (males)	Day 21 (females)	Day 28 (males)	Day 28 (females)	Day 30 (males)	Day 30 (females)
3.5	1 in 5,000	23/28	11/27	24/28	10/26	15/24	8/27
3.7	1 in 10,000	23/28	9/27	24/28	10/26	13/24	7/27
4.0	1 in 32,000	22/28	8/27	24/28	9/26	12/24	5/27
4.5	1 in 340,000	17/28	5/27	19/28	6/26	7/24	3/27

Source: reference 36

Sport (CAS)) going as far as stating that he would be happy to prosecute on the basis of what he had seen and heard, provided the athlete was a "white European man" (because the large majority of volunteers studied came from this ethnic group and the test worked better in men than women). In addition to the need for studies of more ethnic groups, there were other issues identified, such as the possible effect of injury on the test that required more work to optimise the test. Another major issue discussed was the need for development of the IOC's own immunoassays for IGF-I and P-III-P, the two markers selected for the test. The relevant section of the minutes reads:

> Laboratory Development with the recommendation that the IOC develops its own set of specific immunoassays. Not only will this give the IOC control over the worldwide testing procedure but also through licensing it to other sports bodies will be able to use it as an income generator. There is a need to develop monoclonal antibodies in pairs and because we will need a "confirmatory test" this probably means two pairs of monoclonals need developing for each marker. Assay development is fairly straightforward and validation can be assisted and dramatically shortened by the use of existing GH-2000 samples being stored at –70 °C. The IOC should maintain control over these assays and the specific reagents involved. Commercial kit makers change reagents at their own whim and as a result the "reference ranges" can change without warning. This could cause serious problems in the IOC business and would be best avoided by maintaining control over the reagents. There is a potential secure market to justify this. The stability, collection process, storage and transportation of samples have to be investigated and solved. For example – IGF-I is very stable and withstands boiling but it must be shown that collection in the field and transportation to the laboratory does not influence "the test" significantly; even when samples are collected in extremes of heat and cold. Sydney has to attain ISO standards by next September and they have to have all the necessary processes installed and validated. We believe it is possible within the time. Development of IOC assays will also provide a standard and more refined assay than that available commercially.

A whole series of events, however, conspired to delay further work on the marker test for GH. Shortly after the workshop, we received notification from Dr Patrick Schamasch, the IOC Medical Director, that President Samaranch had asked him to inform us that the IOC would advance us a further £1 million (US$2 million) to keep the project team together and the project moving forward. To our extreme disappointment, however, this offer was subsequently suddenly withdrawn before a contract was signed. This was in September 1999, when our bid for "GH-2000 Phase 2" was rejected by the IOC. The project went into limbo and the teams disbanded.

This was a major disappointment, and whatever the reason, one has to question this decision by the IOC that not only prevented the test being ready for the Sydney Olympic Games in September 2000 but also meant that implementation would still not have taken place eight years later.

The EU had a further call for proposals that included an action line on drug abuse in sport, and the multinational GH-2000 Consortium, enlarged by the inclusion of Professor Strasburger's group but this time not including the IOC as a partner (its inclusion was declined by Prince de Merode), was unsuccessful with its application. In an attempt to keep moving on, the EU proposal was immediately resubmitted to the newly formed WADA, which had now been formally placed in charge of research by the IOC. Despite "encouraging noises" from the nascent WADA, the project was considered "too big." This may have been because the application was made too soon after the creation of WADA and before it had a formal structure and budget to cope with research projects of this size. WADA indicated that it was prepared to reconsider a smaller "pilot" (its word) proposal coming just from the United Kingdom, where it reckoned there was enough ethnic diversity to meet the needs of the project. By now, the United States Anti-Doping Agency (USADA) had been firmly established and had sufficient funding to commission GH research, which was high on its list of priorities. It called for proposals and expressed interest in having submissions from outside the United States.

The cut-down and reworked proposal named "GH-2004" was submitted to USADA and later also to WADA, with the authors as joint principal investigators. It aimed to cover the major ethnic and injury issues raised at the IOC Workshop in Rome. Funding was successfully obtained from USADA on Christmas Eve 2002 to allow the research to continue. In the interim between the end of GH-2000 and the start of GH-2004, PHS had retired from his post in London and was appointed as a Visiting Professor at his local University at Southampton, where RIGH (who had previously worked with PHS in London) was a Senior Lecturer in Endocrinology. The GH-2004 project became established at the University of Southampton but continued its close collaboration with Dr Eryl Bassett (University of Kent) and Professor David Cowan (head of the IOC/WADA Laboratory, King's College London).

The project subsequently received supplementary funding from WADA, which was particularly interested in contributing to the funding of the area of ethnic effects.

In parallel with the GH-2004 project, an "Assay Development" collaborative project (originally part of the GH-2000 Phase 2 proposal) aimed at developing two 'in-house' immunoassays for both IGF-I and P-III-P was submitted to USADA by The Institute for Bioanalytics (IBA) in Connecticut (USA). IBA are an assay development company who had been recruited for our unsuccessful bids for GH-2000 Phase 2 to EU and IOC.

IBA were successful in obtaining a grant from USADA but unfortunately underestimated the difficulty of the project. By the time the grant was used up the project had not been completed and consequently USADA lost confidence in IBA and further approaches for funding were unsuccessful.

6.1.2 The GH-2004 project

In order to address the concerns raised at the IOC Rome workshop, the specific aims of the GH-2004 project were:

1   To investigate possible ethnic effects on two markers of growth hormone action:

   –   to develop a reference range for two growth hormone-sensitive markers (IGF-I and P-III-P) in elite athletes;
   –   to study the variability in these markers over time;
   –   to investigate the sensitivity of these markers to growth hormone administration in different ethnic groups;
   –   to investigate the effects of injury on the growth hormone-sensitive markers in different ethnic groups.

2   To validate a test for growth hormone abuse based on the measurement of these two markers, if possible in time for the Athens Olympic Games.
3   To store aliquots of samples (with appropriate documentation) for future use in adding further GH-sensitive markers and validating new assays.

The GH-2004 project undertook further studies of over 300 elite athletes in the post-competition setting to establish whether there were any systematic differences in IGF-I and P-III-P between athletes of differing ethnic backgrounds. This study proved much more challenging to complete than the previous GH-2000 studies. The GH-2004 project manager approached over 60 sporting bodies for permission to undertake this research at their events but permission was granted only at nine events. Following from this, there was resistance from team coaches and doctors, who on occasion specifically refused permission for us to approach their teams.

Even the response rate from the athletes was extremely variable, and we have been disappointed by the small proportion of athletes who have been prepared to volunteer for the study. For example, at the Ninth IAAF World International Athletics Championships in Paris in 2003, only 1 in 30 athletes who were approached agreed to take part in the study. We had greater success in recruiting from smaller events, which tended to have a lower media profile, where the response rate was nearer to 1 in 3 athletes.

It is difficult to understand why the research was so much more difficult to perform only four to five years after the original GH-2000 study, where elite athletes were at times literally standing in line to volunteer. Linguistic and cultural issues may have played a role, but there appeared to an increased feeling of distrust towards the anti-doping agencies, and although we guaranteed anonymity, this may have been a disincentive. We also cannot exclude the possibility that some of the athletes we approached were in fact doping. Certainly one sprinter we approached was subsequently convicted of doping with anabolic steroids.

Despite these difficulties in recruiting as many athletes as we had planned, it was clear that the age effect on marker levels was still apparent in the athletes of differing ethnic background, but there were no major systematic differences in marker concentrations. Although we found minor ethnic differences between groups (for example, the mean IGF-I concentrations in African Caribbean men are approximately 20 percent lower than for white European men), nearly all the values lie within the 99 percent prediction intervals for white European athletes, regardless of ethnic background.

Following the publication of the GH-2000 study results, several other groups in Australia, Japan, Germany, Italy and Spain have undertaken further research to validate the GH-dependent markers approach. One group, led by Professor Ken Ho, has also examined the demographic factors that affect serum IGF-I and P-III-P. Consistent with the results of the GH-2000 and GH-2004 projects, age was found to be the major contributor, accounting for 20.2 percent and 34.3 percent of the variance of IGF-I and P-III-P respectively. In contrast, a further 10 percent and 7 percent of the variance of IGF-I and P-III-P could be explained by gender, sporting discipline, ethnicity and body mass index.

6.1.3 Within-athlete variability

A series of prospective and retrospective studies examining the intra-individual variability of IGF-I and P-III-P have been undertaken in elite and amateur athletes.

ELITE ATHLETES: THE GH-2000 STUDY

Up to four fasting blood samples were obtained from 175 male and 83 female elite athletes over a period of up to one year. The athletes were recruited at national or international sporting events. The vast majority of the athletes were white European, with only 4 African Caribbean and 1 Oriental subject. The mean age of the men and women was 25.9 ± 0.4 yrs and 24.7 ± 0.5 yrs respectively.

The intra-subject variation of IGF-I and P-III-P is illustrated in Figure 10.5. Statistical analysis showed that the intra-individual variation was 14.7 ± 7.0 percent for IGF-I and 14.9 ± 7.0 percent for P-III-P. When the GH-2000 formula was applied to these data, the intra-individual variability of the male formula was 15 ± 4 percent and that of the female formula was 25 ± 6 percent.[38]

ITALIAN ELITE ATHLETES

IGF-I and P-III-P had been previously measured in a longitudinal follow-up study of 25 male and 22 female elite Italian athletes from nine different sporting disciplines.[39,40] The mean ages of the men and women were 22.6 ± 0.2 yrs and 22.5 ± 0.2 yrs respectively. Four blood samples had been taken over a six-month

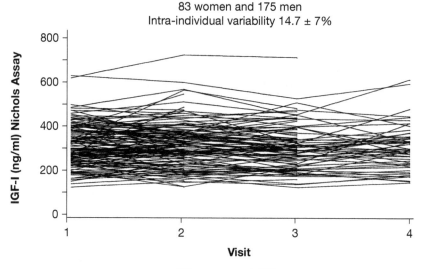

83 women and 175 men
Intra-individual variability 14.7 ± 7%

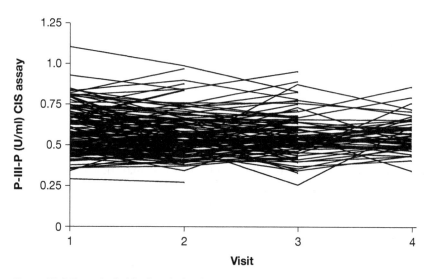

83 women and 175 men
Intra-individual variability 14.9 ± 7%

Figure 10.5 Intra-individual variation in IGF-I and P-III-P in 175 male and 63 female
elite athletes.

period. IGF-I concentrations were determined by using a commercial immunoassay kit (Mediagnost GmbH, Tübingen, Germany). The intra- and inter-assay coefficients of variation were 3.5 percent and 7 percent for IGF-I, respectively. P-III-P levels were determined using the Orion Diagnostica RIA kits (Espoo, Finland). Intra- and inter-assay coefficients of variation were 4.3 percent and 5.3 percent for P-III-P; the sensitivity was 0.2 g/L for P-III-P.

These data were made available to us by the kind permission of Dr Alessandro Sartorio. Our analysis shows that the intra-individual variation in this cohort is consistent with the data from the GH-2000 study (16 ± 8 percent for IGF-I and 18 ± 9 percent for P-III-P).

AMATEUR ATHLETES

The GH-2000 and GH-2004 projects have undertaken two double-blind placebo-controlled GH administration studies.[22,23] In these studies, GH was administered for 28 days and then subjects were followed up for a further 56 days during the wash-out period. During the three-month study, the subjects gave up to seven blood samples in the GH-2000 study and nine samples in the GH-2004 study. The placebo-treated subjects therefore provide us with an opportunity to study the intra-individual variation of IGF-I and P-III-P in amateur athletes. The GH-2000 study included 18 women (24.3 ± 0.9 yrs) and 21 men (26.0 ± 0.9 yrs) who received placebo, all of them white European (the GH-2004 study investigated a more ethnically diverse group). The GH-2004 study included 5 women (23.3 ± 1 years) and 10 men (24.7 ± 1.3 years) who received placebo.

The intra-individual variation was 13.9 ± 7.0 percent and 14.0 ± 7.0 percent for IGF-I in the GH-2000 and GH-2004 studies respectively. The intra-individual variation was 12 ± 6 percent and 19 ± 9 percent for P-III-P in the GH-2000 and GH-2004 studies respectively. When the gender-appropriate GH-2000 formula was applied to the GH-2000 data, the intra-individual variability of the formula in men was 12 ± 2 percent and in women was 25 ± 3 percent.

The results from these four studies show remarkably consistent results, with no apparent difference between amateur and elite athletes. The intra-individual variability for IGF-I varies between 13.9 percent and 16 percent while the variability for P-III-P varies from 12 percent to 19 percent. These data suggest that the sensitivity of a test for GH based on markers might be improved by the concept of an athlete "passport" or "profiling."

6.1.4 GH administration

A further double-blind GH administration study in volunteer amateur athletes undertaken within the GH-2004 project showed that the response to GH in other ethnic groups is similar to that of white Europeans.

6.1.5 Effects of injury

The effect of injury was systemically examined by the GH-2004 team, who followed 143 men and 40 women following a sporting injury. There was no change in IGF-I over the 12-week follow-up, but P-III-P rose by approximately

40 percent, reaching a peak two to three weeks after injury, the magnitude and duration of which varied according to the type and severity of injury. Importantly, however, this did not cause any false positive readings in the proposed test combining IGF-I with P-III-P.

6.2   Other marker approaches

6.2.1   IGF-I/IGFBP2

The ratio of IGF-I to IGFBP-2 in blood has been proposed as a possible method of detecting GH abuse.[34] When rhGH was given at a dose of 0.15 IU/kg subcutaneously for three days to a group of eight healthy young men, it was found that IGF-I and IGFBP-3 rose, while IGFBP-2 fell. The ratio IGF-I/IGFBP2 increased to more than fivefold and remained elevated 30 hours after the last injection of GH.

Although this looked like a very promising approach, the changes in IGFBP-2 in this study were much greater than those seen by the GH-2000 project, where rhGH was administered at the same dose for 28 days. In the GH-2000 studies, the ratio IGF-I to IGFBP-2 did not turn out to be as useful a discriminator of those taking GH as did the combination of serum concentrations of IGF-I and P-III-P.

6.2.2   The Kreischa Study

The Institut für Dopinganalytik und Sportbiochemie (in Kreischa, Germany) undertook a placebo-controlled double-blind GH administration study and developed an alternative discriminant function based on IGF-I and P-III-P but also including IGFBP-3.[41] In this study, 15 young, healthy male amateur athletes were assigned randomly to either placebo or 0.06 IU/kg body weight/day rhGH. Treatment was administered daily by medical staff to the athletes by subcutaneous injection for 14 days, and blood samples were taken for analysis of IGF-I, IGFBP-3 and P-III-P fasting at baseline (day 0) and on days 2, 4, 6, 8, 10, 12, 15 and 18 at 6 p.m.

In order to help validate the GH-2000 formula, Dr Astrid Kniess kindly provided us with a copy of the data from her study. After suitable adjustment for the differences in assay calibration, the GH-2000 formula was applied and was found to detect over 90 percent of those receiving GH with a pre-specified specificity of 1 in 10,000 despite the lower doses of GH used in the Kreischa study.

The Kreischa formula also performed equally well when applied to the data obtained from individuals receiving low-dose GH in the GH-2000 double-blind study. The Kreischa formula performed less well, however, when applied to those receiving high-dose GH and those who had a large increase in markers. This occurs because as P-III-P concentrations rise above a certain figure, the negative product of the term (IGF-I $\times$ P-III-P) leads to a fall in score to below the cut-off point and thus false negative results. This is important because it has been suggested that athletes may be currently receiving up to 10 times higher doses than the amount of GH administered in either the GH-2000 or the Kreischa studies.[42,43] Consequently, the Kreischa function may not be able to detect athletes administering higher GH doses. A further potential disadvantage of the Kreischa formula is the inclusion of IGFBP-3. As anabolic steroids, which are commonly abused with GH, may block the GH-induced increase in IGFBP-3, even when IGF-I is increased significantly, the use of IGFBP-3 in the formula may lower its reliability in detecting the inappropriate use of rhGH in athletes in certain settings.[43]

6.2.3 The Combination of Growth Hormone and Anabolic Steroids

As it is well appreciated that athletes frequently use multiple performance-enhancing drugs, including anabolic steroids, the Australian–Japanese consortium led by Professor Ken Ho has recently completed a study evaluating the effect of co-administration of testosterone and GH in male amateur athletes, and the results show that the additional use of testosterone does not adversely affect the performance of the test.[44]

It is not known how well these GH-2000 formulae will perform in "real life" where the patterns and doses of GH abused by athletes are unclear, but there is now indisputable scientific evidence that should be able to survive legal attack that this method both is feasible and can achieve the detection of athletes receiving GH with both high sensitivity and specificity. The GH-2004 team is currently collaborating with UK Sport in evaluating the marker method within elite sport in the United Kingdom with the expectation that this will facilitate the adoption of the method by WADA.

6.3 The isoform method

The test for GH abuse based on the analysis of GH isoforms was originally termed the "direct method,"[45] but it is now more accurately referred to as the "differential isoform method." Endogenous GH exists in several isoforms, the 22-kD isoform being the most abundant, constituting 75 percent of the circulating GH. The other isoforms are collectively termed "non-22-kD" (including the 20- and 17-kD isoforms and many fragments). Recombinant GH contains only the 22-kD isoform, and exogenous rhGH administration leads by negative feedback mechanisms to a marked decrease in the endogenous pituitary-derived non-22-kD isoforms. Based on this feedback inhibition of endogenous GH secretion, a high ratio of 22- to non-22-kD has been proposed as a mechanism of detecting exogenous rhGH usage (Figure 10.6).[33] Age, sex, physiological stimulus, ethnicity and pathological state have been reported not to affect the relative proportions of GH isoforms. This was shown by the Australian–Japanese consortium, who found that less than 7 percent of the total variability of the log 20 kD:22 kD ratio (measured by the Australian–Japanese

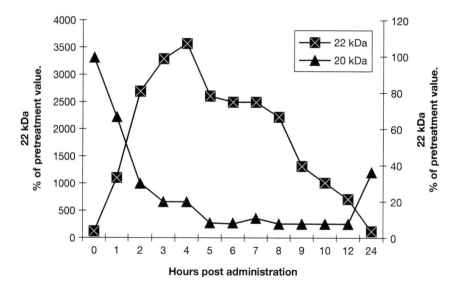

Figure 10.6 Effect of administration of one dose of rhGH on 22-kD and 20-kD isoforms of GH, expressed as a percentage of pretreatment values.

Source: reference 33

method) could be explained by age, BMI, gender, sporting category and ethnicity in Australian elite athletes.

Using assays directed against 22-kD GH and total GH, Strasburger and Bidlingmaier have shown that the ratio between 22-kD and total GH is less than 1, with a normal distribution of values in normal healthy subjects, while individuals receiving GH have values that are greater than 1. Precise sensitivity and specificity are not available for this methodology, although the available data would suggest that a cut-off of around 1.1 would be needed to give a specificity of 1 in 10,000.

It is also unclear how sensitive the test is in relation to rhGH dosage and the "window of opportunity" after the last injection of rhGH when the test can be expected to be positive. Exercise causes a transient relative increase in the 22-kD isoform; therefore, samples taken immediately after competition (the usual scenario) may lower the test's sensitivity.

GH isoforms have half-lives measured in minutes, and for this reason the window of opportunity for detection is short. It has been shown that blood samples taken as soon as 12 hours after a subcutaneous injection of a relatively high dose of rhGH rarely contain measurable amounts of rhGH in women and only low levels (circa 4.5 ng/mL) in men.[46] Thus, the clearance of injected GH is much quicker in women than in men, probably on account of their extra body fat, which contains a high density of GH receptors[47] and because GH clearance is receptor mediated.[48] It has been shown that spontaneous GH secretion returns 48 hours after the last dose of rhGH treatment.[49] The isoform method cannot detect pituitary-derived GH doping (pituitary-derived GH from both animals and humans is still available, particularly on the sport's black market), the abuse of GH secretagogues or IGF-I. Thus, the isoform method is unlikely ever to catch a GH abuser in the classical "post-competition" dope-testing scenario but is more likely to be useful in out-of-competition testing.

As two sets of assays for both 22-kD and total GH had been developed in-house by Strasburger and Bidlingmaier, the problems associated with the use of commercial immunoassays were not applicable to the isoform test, and as a result, WADA and the IOC introduced the isoform method at the Athens and Turin Olympic Games in 2004 and 2006 respectively. As might be anticipated for the reasons just stated, no positives were detected, and indeed it was a minority of samples tested that had a sufficiently high concentration of GH to allow a verifiable test.

This test has been improved and updated and moved from the academic to the commercial world. WADA has commissioned the commercial implementation to allow roll-out to its worldwide network of laboratories. At the time of writing, the new assay kits are currently under evaluation and are expected to be ready for the Beijing Olympic Games in 2008.

The use of immunoassay techniques in forensic toxicology is controversial despite widespread acceptance in laboratory scientific practice.[50] This potential weakness of immunoassays in testing for GH abuse applies equally to the isoform and marker methods but it does seem inconceivable that the final arbiters, the CAS will not accept the best-validated clinical science when they are faced with strong evidence.

An alternative approach to measuring the 22-kD to total GH ratio has been adopted by the Australian–Japanese consortium, which has developed an immunoassay to detect 20-kD. Preliminary data suggest that this is a reasonable alternative to the measurement of total GH.

6.4 Future technologies to detect growth hormone

6.4.1 Surface plasmon resonance

Surface plasmon technology is a non-labelled optical methodology that measures the refractive index of small quantities of a material absorbed onto a metal surface allowing measurement of mass. This technology is being applied to the detection of GH and dependent markers by the Barcelona anti-doping laboratory but at present does not yield the same sensitivity as conventional immunoassays.

6.4.2 Mass spectrometry

Surface-enhanced laser desorption/ionisation time-of-flight mass spectrometry (SELDI-TOF MS) is a proteomic technique in which proteins are bound to proprietary protein chips with different types of adsorptive surfaces. It can be used to analyse peptide and protein expression patterns in a variety of clinical and biological samples, and biomarker discovery can be achieved by comparing the protein profiles obtained from control and patient groups to elucidate differences in protein expression. This technique has been applied to the detection of GH abuse to find potential new markers of GH abuse, such as the haemoglobin α-chain, but the sensitivity is insufficient to deal with analyses of IGF-I and P-III-P.[51]

6.5 Doping with growth hormone secretagogues

The search for an effective oral GH secretagogue has been extensive, but so far none of the potential substances has reached the marketplace. In fact, the development of GH secretagogues seems to have been discontinued by most pharmaceutical companies. The reasons for this are related to the difficulty of designing a secretagogue that has good bioavailability and is entirely specific for GH, combined with the extreme expense of suitable clinical validation and safety trials. The substance that got nearest to the marketplace was MK-0677, a small, orally active molecule that was shown to be a potent secretagogue and to have useful clinical activity in increasing bone mineral density in elderly people[52] and improving rehabilitation after hip fracture.[53] The clinical effects produced were not dramatic, and the costs of running the multinational, multi-centre, double-blind placebo-controlled trials must have been enormous. Thus, it appears that further development was abandoned. The history of GH secretagogue discovery and development is a fascinating story and has been extensively reviewed.[54]

There is still the possibility that existing GH secretagogues will prove to be performance enhancing, and the discovery of this action by athletes and their coaches before the clinical scientists would cause no surprise. After all, their validation trials are much quicker and cheaper, and are probably more sensitive than the massive bureaucratic clinical trials that are now a prerequisite for the launch of a new drug. The abuse of a secretagogue would manifest itself in a manner indistinguishable from that of abuse of GH. The isoform method would be of no use, as the GH secreted by the pituitary would be the usual mixture of isoforms, but the marker method should prove as effective as with the detection of GH injections. As GH secretagogues tend to be relatively small molecules, they may be excreted unchanged in the urine, where they may be readily detected by mass spectroscopy or immunoassay. The finding of even traces of these "foreign substances" would then be an offence.

6.6 Doping with IGF-I

Insulin-like growth factor I (IGF-I; so called because its chemical structure is closely related to that of insulin) mediates a number of actions of GH and is likely to be performance enhancing and a drug of abuse in sport. Its use is banned under the existing WADA and IOC codes. Until recently, IGF-I was in very short supply, and, being a complex molecule, unlikely to be manufactured by anyone other than by a major pharmaceutical company. Recently, two preparations have received FDA approval for clinical use and have become commercially available. One, manufactured by Tercica, is rhIGF-I, identical to the native human hormone. It requires twice-daily injections as it has a short half-life in the body. The other preparation, manufactured by Insmed, consists of rhIGF-I in association with recombinant human IGFBP-3. The advantage of this as a pharmaceutical agent is that its longer half-life in the body means that it requires only once-daily injections. It also produces fewer side effects, particularly hypoglycaemia, at higher therapeutic doses. There is currently a patent dispute between the companies, and at present Insmed is not allowed to market its product in the United States. It is likely that illegal supplies of IGF-I will be available on the "black market," and it is inevitable that supplies will become available from China and "high-tech" underground laboratories elsewhere before long. It is already being promoted on body-building websites.

Detection of IGF-I abuse will provide new problems and challenges, but the marker method being developed for detecting GH abuse should provide a sound scientific basis for a suitable method. WADA has recently approved a research grant to follow up this possibility, but it will be several years before a test will be available.

When IGF-I or IGF-I/IGFBP3 complex is administered to normal people, it stimulates many (if not all) of the anabolic processes stimulated by GH. There is still uncertainty as to the extent to which IGF-I physiologically induces changes attributable to GH. In fact, our knowledge base of the effects of IGF-I in normal subjects is very limited, largely because it is, like insulin, a powerful hypoglycaemic agent. Insulin itself is probably widely abused, and detecting this abuse is extremely difficult.[18] The risks of hypoglycaemia are less with IGF-I, and it is probably a more potent anabolic agent. It acts through stimulating protein synthesis (Figure 10.1) in concert with insulin, which is anabolic through inhibiting protein breakdown. Insulin is more active (and powerful) in the metabolism of glucose than of protein, while the reverse is true for IGF-I.

6.6.1 What are the expected effects of IGF-I abuse on the "marker method"?

IGF-I or IGF-I/IGFBP3 complex administration to normal people inhibits endogenous GH secretion through a normal physiological feedback mechanism. The effects of a single injection are transient, albeit longer with the IGF-I/IGFBP3 complex than with the native unbound hormone. To obtain therapeutic effects, either preparation (like GH) will need to be taken on a regular basis, optimally with daily injections. In order to achieve sufficient change in body composition to enhance performance, weeks if not months of dosing will be required.

The feedback inhibition of GH secretion will lead to a fall in endogenous IGF-I and IGFBP-3 production. IGF-I levels will be lower than normal only for a short period after the injected IGF-I has been cleared and before the pituitary gland has recovered from the feedback inhibition. IGFBP-3 concentration will fall during IGF-I administration as IGFBP-3 production is regulated by GH and takes some time to recover after IGF-I administration stops. IGFBP-2 levels will probably rise during IGF-I administration (compared with a fall with GH) and take a while to recover after IGF-I administration ceases. It is not clear what will happen to other IGF-I binding proteins. Markers of collagen and bone metabolism are expected to rise during IGF-I administration and stay elevated for some time after administration comes to an end.

The above is largely speculation, but forms the basis of the next WADA-funded research project to be undertaken by the GH-2004 team at Southampton University starting in January 2008.

7 Acknowledgements

The origin of GH-2000 occurred at a chance breakfast meeting of PHS with the current president of the IOC, Jacques Rogge. Without his initiative in getting the EU to recognise the importance of research into drug abuse we might not have advanced at all, but we have to ask why the IOC spent more than $1 million of its own money (and much more than $1 million of other people's money) sponsoring its first "commissioned" piece of research only to do nothing with the results?

The authors would like to acknowledge the team effort that has gone into the GH-2000 and GH-2004 projects. Our special thanks go to the rest of the GH-2004 team: Eryl Bassett, Ioulietta Erotokritou-Mulligan, David Cowan, Christiaan Bartlett, Nishan Guha and Cathy McHugh. The GH-2004 study was undertaken in the Wellcome Trust Clinical Research Facility (WT-CRF) at Southampton General Hospital and we acknowledge the support of the WT-CRF nurses and Southampton medical students who have supported the study. It has been a long journey and we are not there yet. It has been a colossal amount of new scientific research, yielding information that might otherwise have remained latent. The level of international collaboration has been a model of what can be done between various national teams who might be considered "scientific rivals." This model of "commissioned" research has been found to be very effective and has delivered a massive amount of invaluable scientific information even if has not been adopted by the IOC and WADA. Thank you to everyone who took part in these projects and thank you to USADA and WADA for continuing the investment.

8 References

1 Li CH, Evans HM, Simpson ME. Isolation and properties of the anterior hypophyseal growth hormone. *Journal of Biological Chemistry*. 1945; 159: 353–66.

2 Raben MS. Treatment of a pituitary dwarf with human growth hormone. *Journal of Clinical Endocrinology and Metabolism*. 1958; 18: 901–3.

3 Raben MS. Growth hormone. 2. Clinical use of human growth hormone. *New England Journal of Medicine*. 1962; 266: 82–6.

4 Duchaine D. *Underground Steroid Handbook*. 1982.

5 Jorgensen JO, Pedersen SA, Thuesen L, Jorgensen J, Ingemann-Hansen T, Skakkebaek NE, Christiansen JS. Beneficial effects of growth hormone in GH-deficient adults. *Lancet*. 1989; 1(8649): 1221–5.

6 Salomon F, Cuneo R, Hesp R, Sonksen PH. The effects of treatment with recombinant human growth hormone on body composition and metabolism in adults with growth hormone deficiency. *New England Journal of Medicine*. 1989; 321: 1797–803.

7 Hintz RLA. The prismatic case of Creutzfeldt-Jakob disease associated with pituitary growth hormone treatment. *Journal of Clinical Endocrinology and Metabolism*. 1995; 80(8): 2298–301.

8 Van Cauter E, Latta F, Nedeltcheva A, Spiegel K, Leproult R, Vandenbril C, Weiss R, Mockel J, Legros JJ, Copinschi G. Reciprocal interactions between the GH axis and sleep. *Growth Hormone and IGF Research*. 2004; 14(Suppl. A): S10–17.

9 McGauley G, Cuneo R, Salomon F, Sonksen PH. Psychological well-being before and after growth hormone treatment in adults with growth hormone deficiency. *Hormone Research*. 1990; 33(Suppl. 4): 52–4.

10 Cuneo R, Salomon F, Wiles C, Hesp R, Sonksen PH. Growth hormone treatment in growth hormone-deficient adults. I. Effects on muscle mass and strength. *Journal of Applied Physiology*. 1991; 70(2): 688–94.

11 Cuneo R, Salomon F, Wiles C, Hesp R, Sonksen PH. Growth hormone treatment in growth hormone-deficient adults II. Effects on exercise performance. *Journal of Applied Physiology*. 1991; 70(2): 695–700.

12 Jorgensen JOL, Thuesen L, Muller J, Ovegen P, Skakkebaek NE, Christiansen JS. 1994. Three years of growth hormone treatment in growth hormone-deficient adults: near normalization of body composition and physical performance. *European Journal of Endocrinology*, 1994; 130: 224–8.

13 Russell-Jones DL, Weissberger A, Bowes SB, Kelly JM, Thomason M, Umpleby AM, Jones RH, Sonksen PH. The effects of growth hormone on protein metabolism in adult growth hormone deficient patients. *Clinical Endocrinology*. 1993; 38: 427–31.

14 Cuneo RC, Salomon F, Watts GF, Hesp R, Sonksen PH. Growth hormone treatment improves serum lipids and lipoproteins in adults with growth hormone deficiency. *Metabolism*. 1993; 42(2): 1519–23.

15 Christ ER, Cummings MH, Westwood NB, Sawyer BM, Pearson TC, Sonksen PH, Russell-Jones DL. The importance of growth hormone in the regulation of erythropoiesis, red cell mass, and plasma volume in adults with growth hormone deficiency. *Journal of Clinical Endocrinology and Metabolism*. 1997; 82(9): 2985–90.

16 Cuneo R, Salomon F, McGauley G, Sonksen PH. The growth hormone deficiency syndrome in adults. *Clinical Endocrinology*. 1992; 37: 387–97.

17 Russell-Jones DL, Bowes SB, Rees SE, Jackson NC, Weissberger AJ, Hovorka

R, Sonksen PH, Umpleby AM. Effect of growth hormone treatment on postprandial protein metabolism in growth hormone-deficient adults. *American Journal of Physiology*. 1998; 37(6): E1050–E1056.

18 Sonksen PH. Insulin, growth hormone and sport. *Journal of Endocrinology*. 2001; 170(1): 13–25.

19 Berggren A, Ehrnborg C, Rosen T, Ellegård L, Bengtsson B-A, Caidahl K. Short-term administration of supraphysiological recombinant human growth hormone (GH) does not increase maximum endurance exercise capacity in healthy, active young men and women with normal GH-insulin-like growth factor I axes. *Journal of Clinical Endocrinology and Metabolism*. 2005; 90: 3268–73.

20 Wallace JD, Cuneo RC, Baxter R, Orskov H, Keay N, Pentecost C, Dall R, Rosen T, Jorgensen JO, Cittadini A, Longobardi S, Sacca L, Christiansen JS, Bengtsson BA, Sonksen PH. Responses of the growth hormone (GH) and insulin-like growth factor axis to exercise, GH administration, and GH withdrawal in trained adult males: a potential test for GH abuse in sport. *Journal of Clinical Endocrinology and Metabolism*. 1999; 84: 3591–601.

21 Wallace JD, Cuneo RC, Lundberg PA, Rosen T, Jorgensen JO, Longobardi S, Keay N, Sacca L, Christiansen JS, Bengtsson BA, Sonksen PH. Responses of markers of bone and collagen turnover to exercise, growth hormone (GH) administration, and GH withdrawal in trained adult males. *Journal of Clinical Endocrinology and Metabolism*. 2000; 85: 124–33.

22 Dall R, Longobardi S, Ehrnborg C, Keay N, Rosen T, Jorgensen JO, Cuneo RC, Boroujerdi MA, Cittadini A, Napoli R, Christiansen JS, Bengtsson BA, Sacca L, Baxter RC, Basset EE, Sonksen PH. The effect of four weeks of supraphysiological growth hormone administration on the insulin-like growth factor axis in women and men. GH-2000 Study Group. *Journal of Clinical Endocrinology and Metabolism*. 2000; 85: 4193–200.

23 Longobardi S, Keay N, Ehrnborg C, Cittadini A, Rosen T, Dall R, Boroujerdi MA, Bassett EE, Healy ML, Pentecost C, Wallace JD, Powrie J, Jorgensen JO, Sacca L. Growth hormone (GH) effects on bone and collagen turnover in healthy adults and its potential as a marker of GH abuse in sports: a double blind, placebo-controlled study. The GH-2000 Study Group. *Journal of Clinical Endocrinology and Metabolism*. 2000; 85(4): 1505–12.

24 Healy ML, Gibney J, Russell-Jones DL, Pentecost C, Croos P, Sonksen PH, Umpleby AM 2003 High dose growth hormone exerts an anabolic effect at rest and during exercise in endurance-trained athletes. *Journal of Clinical Endocrinology and Metabolism*. 2003; 88: 5221–6.

25 Healy ML, Gibney J, Pentecost C, Croos P, Russell-Jones DL, Sonksen PH, Umpleby AM. Effects of high-dose growth hormone on glucose and glycerol metabolism at rest and during exercise in endurance-trained athletes. *Journal of Clinical Endocrinology and Metabolism*. 2006; 91: 320–7.

26 Gibney J, Healy M-L and Sonksen PH. The growth hormone/insulin-like growth factor-I axis in exercise. *Endocrine Reviews*. 2007; 28: 603–24.

27 Hintz RL. 2004. Growth hormone: uses and abuses. Editorial. *British Medical Journal*. 2004; 328: 907–8

28 Rennie MJ. Claims for the anabolic effects of growth hormone: a case of the emperor's new clothes? *British Journal of Sports Medicine*. 2003; 37: 100–5.

29 Giannoulis MG, Sonksen PH, Umpleby M, Breen L, Pentecost C, Whyte M, McMillan CV, Bradley C, Martin FC. The effects of growth hormone and/or

testosterone in healthy elderly men: a randomized controlled trial. *Journal of Clinical Endocrinology and Metabolism*. 2006; 91: 477–84.

30 Graham MR, Baker JS, Evans P, Kicman A, Cowan D, Hullin D, Davies B. Physical effects of short term GH administration in abstinent steroid dependency. *Hormone Research*. 2008; 69: 343–54.

31 Biomedicine and Health (BIOMED 2) 1994–1998. Available from http://cordis.europa.eu/biomed/src/ab-1.htm#1 (accessed January 25, 2008).

32 Biomedicine and Health (BIOMED 2) methodology for the detection of doping with growth hormone and related substances. Available from http://cordis.europa.eu/data/PROJ_BIOMED/ACTIONeqDndSESSIONeq26073200595ndDOCeq4ndTBLeqEN_PROJ.htm (accessed January 25, 2008).

33 McHugh CM, Park RT, Sönksen PH, Holt RIG. Challenges in detecting the abuse of growth hormone in sport. *Clinical Chemistry*. 2005; 51: 1587–93.

34 Kicman AT, Miell JP, Teale JD, Powrie J, Wood PJ, Laidler P, Milligan PJ, Cowan DA. Serum IGF-I and IGF binding proteins 2 and 3 as potential markers of doping with human GH. *Clinical Endocrinology*. 1997; 47(1): 43–50.

35 Healy ML, Dall R, Gibney J, Bassett E, Ehrnborg C, Pentecost C, Rosen T, Cittadini A, Baxter RC, Sönksen PH. Toward the development of a test for growth hormone (GH) abuse: a study of extreme physiological ranges of GH-dependent markers in 813 elite athletes in the postcompetition setting. *Journal of Clinical Endocrinology and Metabolism*. 2004; 90(2): 641–9.

36 Powrie JK, Bassett EE, Sacca L, Christiansen JS, Bengtsson BA, Sönksen PH on behalf of the GH-2000 Project Study Group. Detection of growth hormone abuse in sport. *Growth Hormone and IGF Research*. 2007; 17: 220–6.

37 *GH-2000 Final Report*. Available from http://www.gh2004.soton.ac.uk/GH-2000%20Final%20Report.pdf (accessed January 25, 2008).

38 Holt RIG, Erotokritou-Mulligan I, Cowan DA, Bartlett C, Bassett EE, Muller EE, Sartorio A, Sönksen PH. The GH-IGF-2012 project: the use of growth hormone (GH)-dependent markers in the detection of GH abuse in sport: intra-individual variation of IGF-I and P-III-P. In: Schänzer W, Geyer H, Gotzmann A, Mareck U, eds. *Recent advances in doping* analysis (15), *Proceedings of the Twenty-fifth Cologne Workshop on Dope Analysis*. Cologne: Sport und Buch Strauβ, 2007.

39 Sartorio A, Jubeau M, Agosti F, Marazzi N, Rigamonti A, Muller EE, Maffiuletti NA. A follow-up of GH-dependent biomarkers during a 6-month period of the sporting season of male and female athletes. *Journal of Endocrinological Investigation*. 2006; 29(3): 237–43.

40 Sartorio A, Marazzi N, Sartorio A, Marazzi N, Agosti F, Faglia G, Corradini C, De Palo E, Cella S, Rigamonti A, Muller EE. Elite volunteer athletes of different sport disciplines may have elevated baseline GH levels divorced from unaltered levels of both IGF-I and GH-dependent bone and collagen markers: a study on-the-field. *Journal of Endocrinological Investigation*. 2004; 27(5): 410–15.

41 Kniess A, Ziegler E, Kratzsch J, Thieme D, Muller, RK. Potential parameters for the detection of hGH doping. *Analytical and Bioanalytical Chemistry*. 2003; 376(5): 696–700.

42 Kraemer W, Nindl BC, Rubin MR. Growth hormone: physiological effects of exogenous administration. In: Bahrke MS, Yesalis CE, eds. *Performance-enhancing substances in sport and exercise*. Champaign, IL: Human Kinetics, 2002; 65–78.

43 Karila T, Koistinen H, Seppala M, Koistinen R, Seppala, T. Growth hormone

induced increase in serum IGFBP-3 level is reversed by anabolic steroids in substance abusing power athletes. *Clinical Endocrinology.* 1998; 49(4): 459–63.

44 Nelson AE, Meinhardt U, Hansen JL, Walker IH, Stone G, Howe CJ, Leung KC, Seibel MJ, Baxter RC, Handelsman DJ, Kazlauskas R and Ho KK. Pharmacodynamics of Growth Hormone Abuse Biomarkers and the Influence of Gender and Testosterone: A Randomized Double-Blind Placebo-Controlled Study in Young Recreational Athletes. *J Clin Endocrinol Metab.* 2008; 93: 2213–22.

45 Wu Z, Bidlingmaier M, Dall R, Strasburger CJ. Detection of doping with human growth hormone. *Lancet* 1999; 353: 895.

46 Giannoulis MG, Boroujerdi MA, Powrie J, Dall R, Napoli R, Ehrnborg C, Pentecost C, Cittadini A, Jorgensen, JOL, Sönksen PH on behalf of the GH-2000 Study Group. Gender differences in growth hormone response to exercise before and after rhGH administration and the effect of rhGH on the hormone profile of fit normal adults. *Clinical Endocrinology.* 2005; 62: 315–22.

47 Vahl N, Møller N, Lauritzen T, Christiansen JS, Jørgensen JOL. Metabolic effects and pharmacokinetics of a growth hormone pulse in healthy adults: relation to age, sex, and body composition. *Journal of Clinical Endocrinology and Metabolism.* 1997; 82: 3612–18.

48 Schaefer F, Baumann G, Haffner D, Faunt LM, Johnson ML, Mercado M, Ritz E, Mehls O, Veldhuis JD. Multifactorial control of the elimination kinetics of unbound (free) growth hormone (GH) in the human: regulation by age, adiposity, renal function, and steady state concentrations of GH in plasma. *Journal of Clinical Endocrinology and Metabolism.* 1996; 81: 22–31.

49 Wu RH, St Louis Y, DiMartino-Nardi J, Wesoly S, Sobel EH, Sherman B, Saenger P. Preservation of physiological growth hormone (GH) secretion in idiopathic short stature after recombinant GH therapy. *Journal of Clinical Endocrinology.* 1990; 70: 1612–15.

50 Bowers LD. Analytical advances in detection of performance enhancing compounds. *Clinical Chemistry.* 1997; 43: 1299–304.

51 Chung L, Clifford D, Buckley M, Baxter RC. Novel biomarkers of human growth hormone action from serum proteomic profiling using protein chip mass spectrometry. *Journal of Clinical Endocrinology and Metabolism.* 2006; 91: 671–7.

52 Murphy MG, Weiss S, McClung M, Schnitzer T, Cerchio K, Connor J, Krupa D, Gertz BJ. Effect of alendronate and MK-677 (a growth hormone secretagogue), individually and in combination, on markers of bone turnover and bone mineral density in postmenopausal osteoporotic women. *Journal of Clinical Endocrinology and Metabolism.* 2001; 86: 1116–25.

53 Bach MA, Rockwood K, Zetterberg C, Thamsborg G, Hebert R, Devogelaer JP, Christiansen JS, Rizzoli R, Ochsner JL, Beisaw N, Gluck O, Yu L, Schwab T, Farrington J, Taylor AM, Ng J, Fuh V. The effects of MK-0677, an oral growth hormone secretagogue, in patients with hip fracture. *Journal of the American Geriatrics Society.* 2004; 52: 516–23.

54 Smith RG. Development of growth hormone secretagogues. *Endocrine Reviews.* 2005; 26: 346–80.

11 Gene doping

Theodore Friedmann

1 Genes for treatment of human disease – gene therapy

In the late 1960s, human biology was in the midst of an unprecedented knowledge explosion. Following on the discovery of the structure of DNA by James Watson and Francis Crick in 1953, discovery after discovery followed that began to illuminate the mechanisms by which the DNA genetic information comprising the genes was expressed in both health and disease – how normally functioning genes regulated normal biology and normal human traits, and how defects or "mutations" in the genes were responsible for most human disease – "simple" single-gene genetic diseases such as cystic fibrosis and muscular dystrophy, and complex diseases involving many interacting genetic abnormalities such as most human cancers, diabetes, heart disease and hypertension, Alzheimer's and Huntington's diseases, schizophrenia, etc. It was clear for the first time that these errors were caused by abnormalities in the arrangement of the chemical subunits of DNA – the "bases" "sequence" of DNA – and that the abnormal arrangement of the bases caused the functional products of the genes – the proteins – to have abnormal structures. Such abnormal proteins could no longer perform their vital functions as enzymes, as building blocks of cells, as hormones, etc. and therefore would produce abnormal metabolic effects and disease.

In the late 1960s, medical scientists began to understand that if defective genes were at the heart of so much human disease, a definitive form of treatment of disease could theoretically come about if methods could be developed to correct the abnormalities of the mutant genes themselves, to remove the abnormal genes and replace them with normal genes. This general concept came to be called "gene therapy." In order to develop the methods required for gene therapy, it would be necessary to invent agents that could carry normal foreign genes efficiently into cells in ways that allowed them to produce normal proteins to replace the missing functions causing disease, but as recently as the early 1980s, no such agents were known or readily available. Fortunately, Nature had already invented such agents – that is, viruses. Viruses have evolved to do precisely the job the people interested in gene therapy needed to perform – carry genes into cells and produce new functions in the cells. Of course, normal viruses also needed to develop methods to make many more copies of themselves, and the resulting replication, while beneficial for the virus itself, was not always beneficial for the host that the virus had infected. Out-of-control replication often resulted in disease and even death in the host. But early in the 1980s, gene splicing technology had been invented, and tools suddenly became available to modify the genetic material of the viruses, to remove their deleterious (for the host) genes and replace them with genes of our choice. For example, normal copies of disease-causing genes that might then be transferred into diseased cells and tissue to correct genetic defects and thereby treat and even cure disease. This is an exercise in converting a dangerous biological agent into a disarmed and potentially beneficial and even therapeutic tool – "swords into plowshares."

In 1984, my research group demonstrated that we could indeed use such a modified virus to act as a gene "vector" to introduce a normal gene into cells taken from children with a terrible neurological disease and correct the biochemical defects in the cells. The concept of human gene therapy was born. Soon after this demonstration came a number of additional proofs that foreign genes could indeed correct cell abnormalities of animal models of many other kinds of human disease, and in 1989 the first human clinical study of such an engineered virus was performed at the National Institutes of Health in Bethesda, Maryland. Over the ensuing 16–17 years, numerous human gene transfer studies have been carried out in many countries around the world, and despite a number of serious setbacks and failures, evidence of truly effective treatment of disease in human patients was demonstrated unequivocally in 2002 in small children suffering from genetic causes of abnormally functioning immune systems – the so-called severe combined immunodeficiency diseases (SCID). Even with the best of other forms of therapy, most of these children ordinarily die early in childhood of untreatable infections. But after gene therapy they go to school, play with their friends, roll around in the playground, and require none of the usual antibiotic and other anti-infection treatments – that is, they live normal childhood lives.

Despite the obvious importance of this exciting advance in biomedicine, there is an extremely important cautionary feature. As is true of virtually all other major high-tech areas of clinical medicine, advances come with costs – sometimes very severe ones. Gene therapy is no different. In the same study that demonstrated effective therapy for these little children with life-threatening susceptibility to infections from SCID, four of the 18–19 children treated to date have developed leukemia as a direct result of the treatment. One child has died of his leukemia and the other three are being treated by established anti-leukemia methods. In these cases, we seem to have saved the children from one life-threatening disease only to cause in them a second, equally severe disease. The troubling reality, of course, is that the study is still relatively young and we do not know all of the long-term effects of the treatment. It is possible that additional cases of leukemia or other setbacks will occur. We often accept risks and even known dangers in the cause of doing good – curing disease and relieving suffering – but this need to balance risks and benefits underscores the commonly accepted tenet in the gene therapy community that the technology is still far too immature and potentially dangerous to use in any settings other than serious disease.

There are now many hundreds of gene therapy studies being carried out or being planned in relation to many diseases – among them cancer, degenerative neurological disease, neuromuscular disease.

2 Gene transfer for enhancement?

In the course of performing these therapeutic studies and catalyzed by the growing public recognition of their success and expectations of even more impressive and common successes in the future, it has become clear that the same genetic concepts and tools that are developing and maturing so quickly for the treatment of disease can just as readily be applied to other genetically determined human traits – and of course that leaves out virtually nothing in human biology. The use of biological means to improve already "normal" human traits is no longer "therapy" but is rather an example of "enhancement." And our society already tolerates and even encourages many forms of enhancement: hormone-enhanced growth in normal but small children, cosmetic surgery, drug treatment for inconvenient emotional or cognitive states such as mild neuroses and situational depressions, erectile dysfunction, etc. Indeed, if our society seeks and encourages surgical and drug-based enhancement, it is certainly not difficult to see the advent of gene-based methods for modifying the genetic factors that lead to some of these same traits to give us a functional boost in areas of our lives that we wish to enhance, even though they do not represent diseases or dysfunction.

It is no great surprise that the world of sport has taken notice of the development of gene therapy, and all segments of the sports world – athletes, trainer, regulators – have begun to wonder if the very same concepts and tools that are being developed to cure disease might be used to try to enhance athletic performance. Instead of providing a gene to produce the gene to cure SCID, one can envision attempts to introduce a gene into a muscle or even into the skin of an athlete to produce the hormone erythropoietin in a way that provides an extra and even appropriately controlled increase of red blood cell production when needed in an athletic setting that requires endurance performance. One can imagine methods of genetically enhancing muscle bulk and the power of muscle contraction by providing extra sources of growth hormones or muscle growth factors, not in the form of traditional drugs but rather as genes that can act as introduced as small production factories in some tissue in an athlete.

These approaches are not merely theoretical, but have been demonstrated in animal studies to be feasible and in some cases even efficient. Mice have had additional genes for the muscle growth factor IGF-1 (insulin-like growth factor) introduced into their tissues in ways that produce markedly hypertrophied and powerful muscle. Monkeys and mice have been provided with extra copies of the erythropoietin gene in ways that permit a long-term increase in blood production. But consistent with the safety warning given in the previous section, these methods have proven to be incompletely understood or mastered, and some of the animals expressing increased amounts of erythropoietin, for instance, have developed lethal complications, ironically including complete shutdown of all blood production – untreatable aplastic anemia.

3 An incorrect conventional wisdom

There is a commonly held idea in some scientifically naïve circles that genetic approaches to sports performance enhancement would be undetectable and therefore more attractive to rogue athletes, trainers and others interested in illicit and even dangerous use of this technology. Like so many forms of conventional wisdom, it turns out not to be so very wise. Just as the sophistication of the gene transfer technology itself is increasing, so too is the technology for finding foreign genes and detecting abnormal production of their functional protein products. Both WADA and USADA have instituted major research efforts to apply the powerful tools of modern molecular genetics, including some derived from the wildly successful human genome project, to the detection of gene transfer events. Very encouraging results are coming from those research programs and it is a good bet that methods will become available that are sensitive and specific for gene-based doping and will be no more invasive than currently accepted forms of drug screening and detection.

4 Gene therapy: complex and risk-laden experimental research medicine, not a game

There is no doubt that the concepts and tools of gene therapy will continue to mature and become ever safer. In the therapeutic setting, at the present time this approach to gene transfer is immature, still beset by risks and known hazards and must therefore not be considered mature enough for application in any setting other than ones in which serious disease is being confronted. In those cases, we all generally accept immature technology and expected and even recognized risks. It is a different story with healthy young athletes in which the risk/benefit ratio is heavily in favor of the risk. Trainers or sports physicians who knowingly use the current tools of gene therapy in their athletes should certainly be considered to be guilty of professional misconduct or medical malpractice. Athletes who allow themselves knowingly to be subjected to gene-based doping methods are the victims of their disreputable handlers, misguided, foolish, or all of these.

12 Therapeutic gene use

Jean L Fourcroy

1 Introduction

Gene therapy, better described as gene transfer, is the insertion of genes into an individual's cells and tissues to treat diseases to replace a defective mutant allele with a functional gene. In Chapter 11, Dr Friedmann has given us an excellent overview of the future of gene doping in the world of sports; he has been the leader in this field of gene therapy since the beginning, an important member of the 2002 Symposium on the prospect of gene doping organized by the World Anti-Doping Agency (WADA) and chair of the WADA Gene Doping Panel. He has also been a leader in the oversight of the US trials.[1]

As Dr Friedmann points out in his chapter, it is not a surprise that the world of sport has taken notice of the development of gene therapy.[2] Gene or cell doping is defined by WADA as "the non-therapeutic use of genes, genetic elements and/or cells that have the capacity to enhance athletic perform-ance."[1] New research in genetics and genomics will be used not only to diagnose and treat disease, but also to attempt to enhance human perform-ance.[3] It should be no surprise that athletes might consider the use of genes for its enhancement possibilities. The kinds of genetic modification attractive to sport are well defined: those that stimulate tissue growth, boost strength, and increase stamina by stimulating the production of red blood cells.[4–9]

The discovery of the genetic origin of disease set the stage for the use of gene transfer as therapy.[10] Today, gene therapy research has reached a critical phase and holds great promise to become a widely available form of treatment for disease. The hope is that the introduction of normal genetic material will replace defective genes responsible for a disease or medical problem. There are many diseases that offer the hope of introducing a replacement gene that would continue throughout the person's life to send the constant genetic material to keep muscles in tone, replace hematopoietic cells or prevent cancer.[11–14] Advances in human gene therapy may allow doctors to treat a disease or abnor-mal medical condition by turning off a faulty gene and stopping the growth of a cancerous tumor. Or they may allow the body to begin producing a necessary protein or other substance, such as an enzyme, that the faulty gene cannot order the body to produce.

2 How is a gene transfer achieved?

Gene transfer requires a method of efficiently delivering a functioning gene into the cells of a patient. In recent trials, several different ways have been researched, using carriers to deliver the gene. Major pathways of inserting genetic components are *in vitro*, *ex vivo* and *in vivo*.[10] During *in vivo* gene transfer, the genes are transferred directly into the tissue of the patient. This can be the only possible option in patients with tissues where individual cells cannot be cultured outside the body in sufficient numbers. *In vivo* gene transfer is necessary when cultured cells cannot be reimplanted in patients effectively. During *ex vivo* gene transfer, the cells are cultured outside the body and then the genes are transferred into the cells grown in culture. The cells that have been transformed successfully are expanded by cell culture and then introduced into the patient.

It is almost two decades since that first genetic treatment, on September 14, 1990. Worldwide, researchers have launched more than 400 clinical trials to test gene therapy against a wide array of illnesses, with cancer therapy dominating the field.[11,13,15,16]

3 Who regulates this process?

In the United States, the Food and Drug Administration (FDA) and the National Institutes of Health (NIH) have complementary responsibilities with respect to the regulation of human gene therapy. The FDA's primary job is to make sure that manufacturers produce high-quality and safe gene therapy products, and that these products are properly studied in human subjects. The NIH's primary job is to evaluate both the safety and the quality of the science involved in human gene therapy research.[17–21] Manufacturers of gene therapy products must test their products extensively and meet FDA requirements for safety, purity and potency before they can be sold in the United States. A manufacturer that is considering developing a gene therapy product in the United States first must tell the FDA of its intentions, and then must test the product first in a laboratory and subsequently in research animals. When a manufacturer is ready to study the gene therapy product in humans, it must obtain a special permission exemption from FDA before starting. This exemption is called an investigational new drug application (IND). In the IND, the manufacturer explains how it intends to conduct the study, what possible risks may be involved and what steps it will take to protect patients, and provides data in support of the study. As part of the IND process, the manufacturer also must get approval from a committee of scientific and medical advisers and consumers (called an Institutional Review Board) as well as the Recombinant DNA Advisory Committee (RAC). The RAC is a public advisory committee reporting to the Director of the NIH; it holds regular meetings on gene transfer research and focuses on the scientific, safety and ethical issues involved. RAC members include physicians, scientists, medical ethicists, consumer activists and private citizens, as well as *ex officio* members of the federal government, including employees of the FDA and the Department of Health and Human Services' new Office of Human Research Protection (OHRP).[21–23]

The FDA has not yet approved any human gene therapy product. However, gene-related research and development continues to grow, and the FDA is very involved in overseeing this activity. Since 1989, the FDA has received about 300 requests from medical researchers and manufacturers to study gene therapy and to develop gene therapy products. The number one priority is to have safe human gene therapy studies. It is important to remember that keeping patients safe is not only the government's responsibility. The FDA also expects manufacturers and medical researchers to be responsible and to use the highest-quality experimental products, practice good clinical medicine, and accurately communicate information to FDA and to patients. How to keep current in this field? Fortunately, this is easy since the work of the Office of Biotechnology Activities (OBA) is readily available and transparent.

4 Summary

The safe and effective use of human gene transfer will continue to be a high priority for both the NIH and the FDA. The FDA will strengthen its educational and enforcement programs for manufacturers, spend more time discussing gene therapy with its own staff, organize gene therapy-based research projects, and continue working with the NIH RAC. The world's community of athletic organizations is well aware of these probabilities and the safety concern for our athletes.

5 Acknowledgment

The author thanks Drs D. Hursh and P. Rheistiein for their critical review of the manuscript.

6 References

1 World Anti-Doping Agency, Gene Doping Panel. Available from http://www.wadaama.org/en/dynamic.ch2?pageCategory.id=319 (accessed February 4, 2008).
2 This book, Chapter 11.
3 Unal M, Ozer Unal D. Gene doping in sports. *Sports Medicine*. 2004; 34(6): 357–62.
4 Adams GR. Insulin-like growth factor in muscle growth and its potential abuse by athletes. *British Journal of Sports Medicine*. 2000; 34: 412–13.
5 McCrory P. Super athletes or gene cheats? *British Journal of Sports Medicine*. 2003; 37: 192–3.
6 Miah A. *Genetically modified athletes: biomedical ethics, gene doping and sport*. London: Routledge, 2004.

7 Schneider AJ, Friedmann T. Gene doping in sports: the science and ethics of genetically modified athletes. *Advances in Genetics*. 2006; 51: 1–110.

8 Sweeney HL. Gene doping. *Scientific American*. 2004; 291(1): 62–9.

9 Vogel G. Mighty mice: inspiration for rogue athletes? *Science*. 2004 30 July; 305(5684): 633.

10 Walther W, Stein U. Viral vectors for gene transfer: a review of their use in the treatment of human diseases, *Drugs*. 2000; 60(2): 249–71.

11 Blaese RM. Development of gene therapy for immunodeficiency: adenosine deaminase deficiency. *Pediatric Research*. 1993 January; 33(1 Suppl.): S49–S53.

12 Blaese RM, Culver KW, Miller AD, Carter CS, Fleisher T, Clerici M, Shearer G, Chang L, Chiang Y, Tolstoshev P, Greenblatt JJ, Rosenberg SA, Klein H, Berger M, Mullen CA, Ramsey WJ, Muul L, Morgan RA, Anderson WF. T lymphocyte-directed gene therapy for ADA-SCID: initial trial results after 4 years. *Science*. 1995 October 20; 270(5235): 475–80.

13 Rosenberg SA, Blaese RM, Brenner MK, Deisseroth AB, Ledley FD, Lotze MT, Wilson JM, Nabel GJ, Cornetta K, Economou JS, Freeman SM, Riddell SR, Brenner M, Oldfield E, Gansbacher B, Dunbar C, Walker RE, Schuening FG, Roth JA, Crystal RG, Welsh MJ, Culver K, Heslop HE, Simons J, Wilmott RW, Boucher RC, Siegler HF, Barranger JA, Karlsson S, Kohn D, Galpin JE, Raffel C, Hesdorffer C, Ilan J, Cassileth P, O'Shaughnessy J, Kun LE, Das TK, Wong-Staal F, Sobol RE, Haubrich R, Sznol M, Rubin J, Sorcher EJ, Rosenblatt J, Walker R, Brigham K, Vogelzang N, Hersh E, Eck SL. Human gene marker/therapy clinical protocols. *Human Gene Therapy*. 2000 April 10: 11(6): 919–79.

14 Setoguchi Y, Danel C, Crystal RG. Stimulation of erythropoiesis by in vivo gene therapy: physiologic consequences of transfer of the human erythropoietin gene to experimental animals using an adenovirus vector. *Blood*. 1994; 84(9): 2946–53.

15 Thompson L. Human gene therapy: harsh lessons, high hopes. *FDA Consumer Magazine*. 2000 September–October. Available from http://www.fda.gov/fdac/features/2000/500_gene.html (accessed May 27, 2008).

16 Crystal RG. Transfer of genes to humans: early lessons and obstacles to success. *Science*. 1995; 270(5235): 404–10.

17 Recombinant DNA and Gene Transfer – Office of Biotechnology Activities. Includes *NIH guidelines for research involving recombinant DNA molecules*. Available from http://www4.od.nih.gov/oba/Rdna.htm (accessed February 4, 2008).

18 Human Gene Therapy and the Role of the Food and Drug Administration. Available from http://www.fda.gov/cber/infosheets/genezn.htm (accessed February 4, 2008).

19 Guidance for Industry – Gene Therapy Clinical Trials – Observing Subjects for Delayed Adverse Events. Available from http://www.fda.gov/cber/gdlns/gtclin.htm (accessed February 4, 2008).

20 Cellular and Gene Therapy Publications. Available from http://www.fda.gov/cber/genetherapy/gtpubs.htm (accessed February 4, 2008).

21 Background information on gene therapy clinical trials. Available from http://www.ornl.gov/hgmis/medicine/genetherapy.html (accessed February 4, 2008).

22 US National Institutes of Health recombinant DNA research: notice of intent to propose amendments to the NIH Guidelines for research involving recombinant DNA molecules (NIH Guidelines) regarding enhanced mechanisms for NIH

oversight of recom binant DNA activities. *Federal Register.* 1996 July 8; 61(131): 35774–7.

23 Shipp AC, Patterson AP. The National Institutes of Health system for enhancing the science, safety, and ethics of recombinant DNA research. *Comparative Medicine.* 2003; 53(2): 159–64.

13 Doping and its impact on the healthy athlete

Andrew Pipe

1 Introduction

Increasingly, in the developed world it is a sedentary lifestyle that produces a staggering range of significant health risks, risks that loom large enough to have the potential to decrease the life expectancy of our children.[1,2] In contrast, among a minority of athletes an exceptionally active, competitive lifestyle exposes them to a number of threats to health and well-being. It is important to understand the degree to which sport participation may pose problems to an athlete's physical, emotional and social well-being: involvement in sport may lead to injury, illness and a variety of behavioral and psychological problems. The sport environment, both physical and social, may give rise to a range of problems that have long-term sequelae. In particular – and the focus of this discussion – the abuse of drugs and other prohibited methods for the purpose of enhancing performance threatens both the well-being of sport and the health of athletes. Sport officials, and sport medicine professionals in particular, must be sensitive to the array of problems and issues that may develop in the athletes for whom they care. All in sport have a responsibility to address the dangers posed by doping in a forceful but thoughtful manner.

Three important caveats must be understood. First, the true incidence of the use of prohibited drugs in sport is difficult to define. Second, it is particularly difficult to develop clear evidence of the adverse effects of drugs or compounds whose use is surreptitious; the ability to develop significant clinical experience in defined populations is lacking. Finally, it is naïve in the extreme to believe that a recitation of the side effects of drugs or doping practices, real or potential, will have significant impact in deterring the use of these drugs by individuals who are part of sport subcultures where such drug-taking behavior is the norm or encouraged. It is important that we understand the consequences of such drug-taking behavior; it is equally important that we develop sensitive, realistic and far-reaching programmes to deter this behavior. Ultimately, in my view, it will require nothing less than a cultural shift in many sport environments if we are to be successful.

2 The Prohibited List

Any discussion addressing issues surrounding the use of performance-enhancing drugs must focus first on the substances and products whose use is proscribed in sport. The advent of the World Anti-Doping Agency (WADA) and its Code in 2003 meant that for the first time a universally applied list of forbidden products was applied across an array of sports and nations. The resulting consistency was as welcome as was the more formalized and transparent process used to develop the "Prohibited List."[3,4] The list is assembled on the basis of recommendations emanating from a group of sport clinicians and scientists, which are distributed for comment to stakeholders within the sport community and ultimately ratified by the Executive Committee of WADA. The WADA Code is clear that for a substance to be *considered* for inclusion on the list, it must meet at least two of three criteria: be performance enhancing; injurious to health; or contravene the "spirit of sport". Many fail to apprehend that meeting two of these three criteria does not mean that a substance is automatically placed on the List: water can enhance performance, and in large quantities can contribute to hyponatremia and death, but it would be absurd to add it to the List! The List is reviewed annually and is released to the sport community in the autumn of the year; it becomes active on 1 January of the following year. Substances are categorized carefully, and the List identifies drugs prohibited at all times as well as those prohibited only in competition.

As the list has evolved, so too has the perverse ingenuity of those who seek accentuated performance at any cost. In 2007, the List now specifically identifies "gene doping" as prohibited, in anticipation of the application of gene manipulation in the future; the development of hormonal products as a result of the application of recombinant technology now means that products like the erythropoietins are prohibited; manipulation of other blood products has required the prohibition of intravenous techniques and equipment. The advent of new approaches to doping has been accompanied by the emergence of new, often unanticipated, consequences of doping behavior. At the same time, it is recognized that the legitimate health needs of many athletes frequently require the use of otherwise prohibited medications. The WADA Code provides for the administration of such medications following special application and a review of a particular case by a suitably qualified panel. The inclusion of many very commonly used medications (e.g. β_2-agonists for the treatment of asthma, glucocorticosteroids for the treatment of a variety of inflammatory disorders) has attracted controversy and has also meant that large numbers of applications for permission to use such medications must be processed by sport authorities.

In the paragraphs and pages that follow, the health consequences that may befall athletes who consume prohibited substances will be examined . . . albeit in a cursory fashion. The actual incidence of side effects or adverse consequences of doping activity is unknown. Much of the information surrounding any discussion of these matters is gleaned largely from isolated case reports which probably underrepresent the true incidence of problems. At the same time, it has been noted that the incidence and prevalence of severe side effects are probably small.[5] The discussion will be ordered, in a general sense, according to the categories of the WADA Prohibited List.

3 Anabolic agents

Developed during the Second World War for military reasons, the anabolic agents were introduced to the sport community in the postwar years. Their spread, initially into the subcultures of weightlifting and field events in athletics, was rapid. In almost any sport in which strength and power are important, the potential for anabolic steroid use can be found. Similarly, the development of muscle mass and a certain body-build has led large numbers of young men and women, outside of competitive sport, to use these products – so-called "body image" users.[6,7] As in all areas of health promotion, "scare tactics" designed to minimize or eliminate steroid and other performance-enhancing drug use have proven largely ineffective in changing behavior; programmes that have used an empathic educational approach have seemed more successful in transforming adolescent behaviour.[8] It has been estimated that nearly 30 percent of steroid users experience mild subjective adverse effects.[9] Nevertheless, many steroid users report an enhanced level of energy and sense of well-being, and are pleased with the perceived changes in performance that accompany the use of these drugs.[10–12] Such perceptions accentuate the challenge of counseling against their use.

It is most important to emphasize once again that there have been no clearly defined populations of users from whom might be developed a more comprehensive understanding of the consequences of steroid administration; such administration is illicit and there is almost a complete absence of authoritative clinical experience derived from the systematic follow-up of steroid-using populations. For many years, the clinical community was skeptical of the ergogenic properties of these compounds – much to the amusement of those who were using those products. Only in the late 1980s did clinical authorities concede that these compounds were capable of enhancing strength.[9] It was not until 1996, arguably more than 50 years after the introduction of these drugs, that evidence of their efficacy in increasing muscle mass and strength was clearly established.[13] Anabolic steroids are both anabolic (encouraging the "buildup" of muscle) and androgenic (making masculine). As a consequence, the potential problems associated with their use reflect the side effects of the anabolic processes they engender, the consequences of their masculinizing properties, and a range of other, often unanticipated, physiological consequences.[14] At the same time, it has been noted that these products also exert an influence on the central nervous system so as to produce changes in behavior and enhanced aggressiveness.[15] The reader is directed toward a number of excellent reviews of the clinical and pathological sequelae of steroid use.[16–21]

Anabolic steroids exert their effect by binding to androgen receptors in muscle and other tissue, potentiating protein synthesis within the specific tissue. Specific effects will be produced, dependent on the tissues so stimulated. Anabolic steroids also have an anti-catabolic effect, and, as noted above, may induce a heightened state of arousal and aggressiveness that facilitates prolonged training and enhances recovery.

The use of anabolic androgenic steroids (AAS) can be associated with a variety of adverse effects that are generally thought to be dose related and reflect the variety of systems and tissues influenced by the drugs. Orally ingested anabolic agents travel to the liver, where "first-pass" metabolic processes occur. A variety of hepatic consequences of anabolic steroid use have been postulated and described: elevated liver enzymes may occur in many users (although such enzyme elevations have been noted in non-steroid-using athletes), and several reports of hepatic adenomas in steroid users have appeared over the past 30 years.[22–26] An almost unique consequence of the administration of anabolic steroids, peliosis hepatis, the developments of blood-filled sacs within the liver, has been described in many case reports.[27–30]

Cardiovascular consequences of the use of anabolic agents have been reported on many occasions; once again, an absence of sustained clinical experience with AAS administration in a defined population using similar products and dosing strategies means that much of our information is derived from case reports. Significant alterations in lipoprotein levels (decreased HDL and increased LDL) have been identified.[31–35] Alteration of normal vascular reactivity via diminished endothelial vasodilator function has also been considered a consequence of AAS use.[33,36] Other investigators have examined the effect of AAS on coagulation: some products appear to increase plasminogen activator activity, suggesting a protective effect, while others appear to have activity favouring coagulation.[37,38] The risk of cardiac disease has been estimated to be elevated threefold among those who use AAS.[33,36] Not surprisingly, therefore, the incidence of premature or unanticipated cardio- and cerebrovascular events in athletes is reflected in the numbers of case reports describing such catastrophes.[39–47] Superimposed upon a distorted and potentially atherogenic lipoprotein profile, the dramatic intermittent elevations in blood pressure reported in weight lifters and bodybuilders may also play a role in the development of cerebrovascular accidents in such athletes.[48–50] Changes in the size and structure of the myocardium have also been attributed by a number of authors to AAS use.[51,52] Ventricular dysfunction has been described after long-term misuse of steroids.[53] The development of cardiomyopathy in athletes, and its associated complications, has also been linked to AAS use.[54–56]

In recent years, considerable attention has been paid to the array of behavioral changes associated with the use of AAS.[19] A flourishing literature attests to the range and significance of these effects, which have implications for the community well beyond the precincts of organized sport. Such changes are usually associated with dose and include a spectrum of disorders including depression, mania, psychosis, delirium, and aggressive and homicidal behavior.[57–62] The role of AAS in creating heightened levels of aggression leading to impulsive, violent or self-destructive behavior continues to be the focus of examination by psychiatric and forensic researchers.[62–64] Such behavior frequently affects the families and partners of steroid users.[65–67] Several investigators have described the development of dependence in steroid users – findings that add to the challenge of eliminating their use.[68–72] The recognition and treatment of anabolic steroid dependence is now the focus of clinicians in a few centers.[73,74]

AAS use has been identified as causing an array of other predictable side effects as a consequence of its androgenic properties. Acne, a product of androgen excess, is common in steroid users.[75] In women, the administration of AAS will, in addition to enhancing muscle size, strength and power, contribute to the development of a deeper voice, male-pattern baldness, hirsutism, changes to the genitalia, menstrual irregularities and a coarsening of facial features.[21] In both sexes, AAS will have an impact on reproductive function. Testicular atrophy, oligospermia or azoospermia, and prostatic hypertrophy may occur in men.[76–78] A common consequence of the use of some AAS is the development of gynecomastia: as a consequence of the peripheral conversion of excess androgens to estrogens, the growth of breast tissue is stimulated.[5,79] The use of tamoxifen, an estrogen blocker, is common among many users of AAS who seek to combat or control these developments.[79] Consequently, tamoxifen is now a prohibited drug in sport.

Ironically, muscle growth and strength, under the influence of AAS, may outstrip the strength of tendons, leading to several reports of tendon rupture in steroid users.[80–82] The growth of long bones may be arrested in immature athletes as a consequence of the impact of AAS in fusing the epiphyseal growth plates.[81]

Repeated injections of AAS can lead to infection and abscess formation at the injection sites. The sharing of needles by steroid users poses particular risk of the transmission of infectious diseases such as hepatitis and HIV – a risk that went largely unappreciated until it became clear that large numbers of adolescents in North America were self-administering steroids, and sharing needles in the process.[83,84]

4 Hormones and related substances

As the ability to synthesize a variety of hormones has evolved, so too has the tendency of misguided athletes and sport officials to abuse the products of such scientific progress. The availability of synthetic erythropoietin (rhEPO) and human growth hormone (hGH) pose particular problems for sport and medical authorities while exposing athletes to significant risk.

4.1 Erythropoietin

Erythropoietin, the natural stimulus for the production of red blood cells, is normally produced in the kidneys and exerts its influence on the bone marrow.

The development of rhEPO is a boon for patients with significant hematological, renal or oncologic disorders. Sadly, its ability to increase the production of red blood cells, with a resulting increase in aerobic capacity, has spawned widespread use of the product in a variety of sport cultures.[85] Disastrous results for the health of athletes and the integrity of sport have followed.[86–88]

An increase in the red blood cell count invariably leads to an increase in blood viscosity and therefore may predispose to augmented clotting, which in turn may lead to the development of a variety of thrombotic complications including stroke, myocardial infarction and venous thromboembolism.[89] The abuse of rhEPO in athletic settings, where dehydration is commonplace, may potentiate the likelihood of such untoward events.[90] A significant number of deaths are reported to have occurred in cycling since the commercial availability of rhEPO in the late 1980s. The deaths have been imputed to the use of this hormonal product and its potential to induce thrombotic events.[86] More insidious is the development of "red cell aplasia," a life-threatening complication associated with the use of rhEPO, and the result of the development of antibodies to erythropoietin, with a consequent arrest of red cell production.[91] Finally, concerns are now emerging regarding the relationship between the use of rhEPO and the development of malignant tumors which themselves may be dependent upon the availability of blood supply.[92]

The use of rhEPO was preceded by "blood doping," a process in which the blood of an athlete (an autologous transfusion), or of others (a homologous transfusion), was infused so as to increase the red cell mass. Not surprisingly, such administration was fraught with problems, including transfusion reactions.[93,94] The practice of blood doping declined, it is assumed, with the availability of rhEPO. Sadly, now that technologies are available which make possible the detection of rhEPO, it is believed that the administration of previously collected red blood cells is increasing.

4.2 Human growth hormone

For many years, it has been assumed that human growth hormone (hGH), responsible for stimulating the growth of all body tissues, would confer significant anabolic advantage on those who might have access to this product. Originally derived from cadaver pituitary glands and available in only small amounts for the use of growth deficiency in children, the hormone acquired a reputation within certain sport circles as being a very powerful modifier of strength and power. Use of the cadaver-derived product ceased with the recognition that it could transmit the agent responsible for Creutzfeldt-Jakob disease, a degenerative brain disorder. The advent of a synthetic version of this hormone (recombinant human growth hormone, rhGH), though a boon for the treatment of those with growth deficiency, introduced new challenges for sport authorities as ill-intentioned athletes and others sought to use this product to enhance growth and performance. Growth hormone elicits its responses not by a direct stimulation of target tissues but rather by the production within the liver of insulin-like growth factor (IGF-I). The evidence that hGH is capable of inducing anabolic responses in athletes continues to be debated.[95–98] Nevertheless, there is consensus that the use of this hormone can contribute to an array of adverse effects – best considered by examining those patients with acromegaly, a clinical condition caused by the increased production of natural growth hormone as a result of a pituitary disorder. Such patients are prone to develop a number of problems including high blood pressure, diabetes, cardiomyopathy, coarsened facial features, arthralgias and abnormal lipid metabolism.[99] Increased muscle bulk and strength are not features of the acromegalic syndrome.

4.3 Gonadotrophins

The gonadotrophins (luteinizing hormone (LH) and human chorionic gonadotrophin (hCG)), which possess the ability to induce hormonal activity within the gonads (testes and ovaries), have typically been abused by individuals consuming anabolic steroids, in an attempt to maintain normal testicular function. The use of hCG is intended to mask the intake of anabolic steroids, or to maintain normal testicular function following prolonged anabolic steroid intake with a resulting decrease in testicular activity. It is also the case that the use of hCG will cause an elevation of blood testosterone levels in males with, it may be concluded, a resultant increase in strength.[100] It is difficult to document the adverse consequences of hCG administration to athletes, given the surreptitious nature of such drug usage; concerns have arisen concerning the use of this compound in the treatment of young boys with undescended testes and the subsequent development of deleterious consequences for testicular function.[101,102] Such concerns about the consequences of hCG administration are reflected in the detection of disordered testicular function in athletes using anabolic steroids and hCG.[103]

4.4 Insulin

A principal function of insulin is to facilitate the delivery of glucose into muscle and other cells. This fundamental physiological reality has been misconstrued by some athletes who believe that the administration of insulin will therefore enhance muscle cell growth and strength. This has led to the bizarre and dangerous use of insulin in some sport settings – with predictable consequences.[104] Insulin causes a significant reduction of blood sugar and hypoglycemia; coma and death can follow its inappropriate use.[105–107] The incidence of these phenomena occurring in a sport context is very likely underreported.

5 β$_2$-agonists

The use of β$_2$-agonists, commonly employed to treat asthma, exercise-induced asthma (EIB) or exercise-induced bronchospasm (EIB), is controlled in sport. It is acknowledged that there has been a dramatic increase in the incidence of asthma and related conditions in the past decade, especially in the developed world, and particularly among athletes in a variety of sport disciplines.[108–114] The public health significance of recognizing, and treating, these conditions is significant; asthma is no longer a rare cause of sudden death among active individuals.[112] The most common approach to the treatment of these conditions is the use of β_2-agonist medications, which cause a dilation of the airways. While there is no strong evidence of the ability of most of these products to enhance performance, or of adverse health impacts associated with their use or misuse, they have been prohibited in sport. Permission for their use is obtained by applying to sport authorities for an "Abbreviated TUE,"[3] which is activated following its receipt. A concern has been raised that the use of such medications may contribute to tolerance; these concerns would appear to be unjustified.[115,116] Others have expressed concern about an increased incidence of cardiac side effects in those using β_2-agonists over a period of many years.[117,118] Of more significance is the recognition that reliance on β_2-agonist therapy to maintain control of asthma in the face of worsening symptoms is highly inappropriate – and potentially very dangerous. To ignore changing symptomatology is to court disaster. An asthmatic athlete must monitor their condition carefully, recognizing that declining control is generally indicative of the need for the use of inhaled corticosteroids – now seen as the mainstay of the long-term treatment of asthma. (Inhaled corticosteroids also require an "Abbreviated TUE.") The use of long-term inhaled corticosteroids, particularly among young patients, has raised questions about the impact of these medications on bone health and general growth and development. However, it is generally conceded that the supervised use of inhaled corticosteroids is safe.[119,120]

6   Diuretics and masking agents

In sports where competition is ordered by weight (e.g. rowing, judo, boxing), it has not been unusual for athletes to attempt to "make weight" by employing a variety of bizarre, dangerous practices including forced sweating, food and fluid restriction, and diuretic and laxative abuse. Despite evidence that performance is almost always adversely affected by such practices, the power of sporting dogmas and the influence of sport subcultures are sufficiently pervasive that these practices persist. Diuretics have also been abused in attempts to "flush" prohibited substances from the body, or in ill-conceived attempts to mask their presence. Modern analytical techniques are such that these maneuvers are virtually guaranteed to be unsuccessful. But an athlete who consumes diuretics, for whatever reason, jeopardizes fluid and electrolyte balance, with potentially dangerous consequences ranging from dehydration and collapse to cardiac arrest. These dangers are magnified when competition is taking place in hot, humid conditions.[121] Ironically, there is little evidence to support the contention that performance is enhanced following diuretic-induced dehydration.[122–124]

7 Stimulants

It is impossible to categorize all of the stimulants that could conceivably be abused in sport, let alone identify a list of their side effects and the potential adverse consequences of their use. Stimulant use is prohibited "in-competition," a consequence of the recognition that many "over-the-counter" medications contain decongestant and other agents that are themselves stimulants. Changing tolerance for the incidental use of such medications (given little evidence of their efficacy and the ease with which some of them may form the basis of the clandestine production of amphetamine-related compounds) may serve to limit their availability in the future; pseudoephedrine is a case in point. In the past, caffeine was prohibited when found in the urine above a certain level; it is no longer prohibited, but sport authorities continue to monitor its appearance in doping control samples. Ephedrine, for many years a constituent of many herbal medications and dietary supplements, but no longer commonly used in clinical medicine (and removed from supplements), remains on the prohibited list.

7.1 Amphetamines

In the late eighteenth century, sport's first doping-related death occurred in cycling in association with the use of strychnine, a nonspecific central nervous system stimulant; several other strychnine-related deaths occurred in ensuing years. It was the death in the 1960 Olympic Games of Knut Jensen, a Danish cyclist, followed by the equally tragic death of the British cyclist Tommy Simpson in the Tour de France of 1967, that drew the world's attention to the use of amphetamines in sport. Both of these athletes were discovered to have been using amphetamines – stimulants that had been developed in the early 1920s. As a consequence of these tragedies, the first drug testing in an Olympic Games environment took place in Mexico in 1968 – and amphetamines were the focus of that testing. These powerful stimulants have been used by unscrupulous athletes and their handlers for many years; their ability to enhance certain sport performances has been understood for decades.[125,126] The ability of amphetamines to induce a variety of significant complications has also been known for more than three-quarters of a century.[127] Given the lack of any reference populations, it is always difficult to evaluate patterns of clandestine drug use in sport, but it would seem likely that amphetamine use in competition has declined (the ability to detect the presence of amphetamine combined with the ubiquity of in-competition testing is perhaps responsible for this positive development). Ironically, it may be the case that the "recreational" use of amphetamine-related drugs such as MDMA ("ecstasy") and cocaine have increased as these drugs have become more commonly ingested in social settings (e.g. "raves") that may be attractive to athletes.[128] Irrespective of the mode, or place, of administration, these drugs present very specific hazards to the user as a consequence of their impact on the central nervous, cardiovascular and thermoregulatory systems in particular. Deaths due to disordered thermoregulation, myocardial infarctions and cerebrovascular accidents (strokes) have been well documented in the clinical literature. A growing body of evidence supports the contention that the abuse of amphetamine-related drugs can result in significant psychiatric and neuropsychological morbidity.[127,129–131] But other stimulants are, or were, far more likely to be encountered or abused by athletes.

7.2 Ephedrine

The popularity of nutritional supplements within the athlete community meant that for many years these largely unregulated products frequently contained quantities of ephedrine, a sympathomimetic that was touted to enhance performance, minimize the development of fatigue and facilitate weight loss.[132] It was also a substance whose use resulted in a significant number of deaths in the sport and exercising community because of its propensity, in susceptible individuals, to cause coronary artery spasm, leading to heart attacks and death.[133–140] Other significant side effects are associated with the use of ephedrine and ephedrine-like substances: high blood pressure, tachycardia, tremor and restlessness are commonly associated with these products.

7.3 Cocaine

Cocaine has been described as "the most potent stimulant of natural origin."[141] In use for centuries, the drug has been used to combat fatigue and, more recently, as a "recreational" stimulant. The drug can be inhaled, injected or smoked; irrespective, this drug poses great risk to any user, principally because of its ability to cause pronounced constriction of the coronary arteries with a resulting risk of heart attack and/or sudden death.[142–145] Sadly, the use of this drug became commonplace in certain sport subcultures – until highly publicized deaths of young athletes served to inform others of the hazards implicit in its use. Ironically, despite sensations to the contrary, cocaine use is unlikely to accentuate athletic performance. What can be assured is that use of cocaine carries a high risk of addiction and can lead to a variety of other untoward effects, including changes in neuropsychological, renal, pulmonary, gastrointestinal and otolaryngological function; loss of memory; paranoia; and anxiety.[146–148]

No discussion of stimulant use in sport would be complete without mentioning that the stimulant medications used to treat attention deficit hyperactivity disorder (ADHD) because of their ability to stimulate inhibitory centers of the brain – and thereby produce a quieting, or slowing of otherwise erratic, unfocused behaviors – are prohibited in sport.[149,150] Their use requires a therapeutic use exemption (TUE).

8 Narcotics

The use of narcotic medications to blunt the pain and discomfort of injury or exhaustion was perhaps commonplace in the past. Fortunately, it has been recognized that narcotics depress and sedate – and therefore are highly unlikely to enhance performance. Nevertheless, these drugs are prohibited for very understandable reasons. In certain cases, their use is permitted when treatment of a legitimate clinical condition results in an application for a TUE, which is then carefully reviewed before being granted. Those using narcotics for pain control typically experience a variety of side effects, including constipation, nausea, diminished cognition and respiratory depression.[151]

9 Cannabinoids

The use of cannabinoids (hashish, marijuana) is prohibited in sport. There is little evidence to suggest that these compounds can enhance performance; their sedating properties would tend to be ergolytic in most sporting contexts. Some would argue that the use of cannabinoids is a conduct, not a doping, issue. The consequences of regular cannabinoid use are understood and include a likelihood of dependence and other drug use, diminished academic performance, impaired memory and cognition, "problematic behaviors," and various psychological health problems.[152–154] An understanding has developed, too, of the role of marijuana smoking in producing changes in lung function.[155,156]

10 Glucocorticosteroids

Commonly used around the world in a variety of forms for the treatment of a multiplicity of conditions and disorders (generally involving inflammation or an allergic response), the glucocorticosteroids have been abused by athletes in certain sports where their systemic administration has been noted.[88] Such use is unlikely without the involvement of physicians, trainers and other support personnel. At the same time, the frequent use of these medications in the treatment of athletic injuries has drawn recent careful scrutiny.[157,158]

The systemic administration (via injection or oral administration) of corticosteroids exposes athletes to significant risk, given the role that these compounds can play in suppressing normal physiological responses and in initiating a large number of predictable and highly undesirable side effects. Virtually every organ system can be influenced by corticosteroid therapy: blood, muscles, skin, bone, heart, eyes, brain, gut, and multiple elements of the endocrine system can all be affected.[120,159–163] Only the most irresponsible practitioner would consider administering systemic corticosteroids to an athlete in the absence of any clinical indication to do so.

11 The vulnerability of athletes

It is a unique privilege to be able to care for athletes. The opportunity to provide them with clinical support and a scientific perspective as they seek to improve themselves and their performances is accompanied by very special responsibilities ... to the athlete, to sport, and to the community, which generally, and generously, supports sport activity. The role and responsibility of the sport medicine professional is no different than that of a health professional in any other setting: to provide care of the highest standard, in a manner that is in accord with established codes of professional and ethical conduct. Athletes who happen to be patients are still, first and foremost, patients. As such, they merit the best of care delivered in a manner that reflects, and respects, their unique circumstances and the settings in which they train and compete. Athletes are particularly vulnerable. They are easy prey for the quack and the charlatan ... or even for those who with the best of intentions advocate some new-found, but unproven, approach or therapy.

Sport, and associated training and performance pressures, may reveal or exacerbate existing tendencies in certain athletes. Athletes may be vulnerable to exploitation in a number of ways that have health implications. Many athletes place an inordinate amount of trust in coaches and others in their sport environment; that trust may be abused. An athlete may be seen as a "commodity" to be exploited by family, coaches or the sport organization. Athletes may be exposed to unacceptable risks in the practice of their sport with no ability to anticipate or understand the associated implications. Ironically, athletes may be exposed to substandard or unconventional approaches to the care of illness or injuries as a consequence of the degree to which the dogma or "traditions" of a particular sporting culture influence or dictate the provision of treatment. The current preoccupation with avid intravenous fluid transfusion during training or competition in certain sports (e.g. wrestling, and track and field) is typical of the way in which certain "fads" emerge in sport; ironically, the evidence of the superiority of oral rehydration continues to grow.[164,165]

The pursuit of sporting success may cause young athletes to move away from their family at a very young age. The resulting family disruption and associated social and educational disturbances may have significant long-term impact on the life and well-being of the athlete. Immersion in a narrowly focused sporting world may distort perspectives and alter educational and career aspirations; development in the broadest sense may suffer.

12 Safeguarding the health and well-being of the athlete

If we are to ensure, to the extent possible, the health of athletes, it is essential that they be provided with comprehensive, high-quality health care and sport science support; and they should be protected from bizarre or unsafe practices and approaches to training. Appropriate attention should be paid to injury prevention and the creation of practice and competition environments that are safe. Athletes need advocates: individuals who will act in an athlete's best interests while appreciating their unique aspirations; individuals who understand that their first responsibility is to safeguard the athlete's health and well-being. The sport medicine professional and the sport scientist must exercise those responsibilities at all times.

13 References

1 Blair SN, Kohl HW III, Paffenbarger RS Jr, Clark DG, Cooper KH, Gibbons LW. Physical fitness and all-cause mortality: a prospective study of healthy men and women. *Journal of the American Medical Association.* 1989; 262(17): 2395–401.

2 Olshansky SJ, Passaro DJ, Hershow RC, Layden J, Carnes BA, Brody J, Hayflick L, Butler RN, Allison DB, Ludwig DS. A potential decline in life expectancy in the United States in the 21st century. *New England Journal of Medicine.* 2005; 352(11): 1138–45.

3 WADA. World Anti-Doping Code, version 2.0. Montreal: World Anti-Doping Agency. Available from http://www.wada-ama.org/rtecontent/document/code_v3. pdf (accessed November 16, 2007).

4 WADA. The 2008 Prohibited List International Standard. Montreal: World Anti-Doping Agency, 2007. Available from http://www.wada-ama.org/rtecontent/ document/2007_List_En.pdf (accessed November 16, 2007).

5 Wu FC. Endocrine aspects of anabolic steroids. *Clinical Chemistry.* 1997; 43(7): 1289–92.

6 Wagner JC. Abuse of drugs used to enhance athletic performance. *American Journal of Hospital Pharmacy.* 1989; 46(10): 2059–67.

7 Windsor R, Dumitru D. Prevalence of anabolic steroid use by male and female adolescents. *Medicine and Science in Sports and Exercise.* 1989; 21(5): 494–7.

8 Goldberg L, Elliot D, Clarke GN, MacKinnon DP, Moe E, Zoref L, Green C, Wolf SL, Greffrath E, Miller DJ, Lapin A. Effects of a multidimensional anabolic steroid prevention intervention: the Adolescents Training and Learning to Avoid Steroids (ATLAS) program. *Journal of the American Medical Association.* 1996; 276(19): 1555–62.

9 Haupt HA, Rovere GD. Anabolic steroids: a review of the literature. *American Journal of Sports Medicine.* 1984; 12(6): 469–84.

10 Freinhar JP, Alvarez W. Androgen-induced hypomania. *Journal of Clinical Psychiatry.* 1985; 46(8): 354–5.

11 Pope HG Jr, Katz DL. Affective and psychotic symptoms associated with anabolic steroid use. *American Journal of Psychiatry.* 1988; 145(4): 487–90.

12 Pope HG Jr, Katz DL. Psychiatric and medical effects of anabolic-androgenic steroid use. A controlled study of 160 athletes. *Archives of General Psychiatry.* 1994; 51(5): 375–82.

13 Bhasin S, Storer TW, Berman N, Callegari C, Clevenger B, Phillips J, Bunnell TJ, Tricker R, Shirazi A, Casaburi R. The effects of supraphysiologic doses of testosterone on muscle size and strength in normal men. *New England Journal of Medicine.* 1996; 335(1): 1–7.

14 American Academy of Pediatrics. Committee on Sports Medicine and Fitness. Adolescents and anabolic steroids: a subject review. *Pediatrics*. 1997; 99(6): 904–8.

15 Clark AS, Henderson LP. Behavioral and physiological responses to anabolic-androgenic steroids. *Neuroscience and Biobehavioral Reviews*. 2003; 27(5): 413–36.

16 Ellender L, Linder MM. Sports pharmacology and ergogenic aids. *Primary Care: Clinics in Office Practice*. 2005; 32(1): 277–92.

17 Maravelias C, Dona A, Stefanisdou M, Spiliopoulou C. Adverse effects of anabolic steroids in athletes: a constant threat. *Toxicology Letters*. 2005; 158: 167–75.

18 Thiblin I, Petersson A. Pharmacoepidemiology of anabolic androgenic steroids: a review. *Fundamental and Clinical Pharmacology*. 2004; 19: 27–43.

19 Trenton AJ, Currier GW. Behavioural manifestations of anabolic stereoid use. *CNS Drugs*. 2005; 19(7): 571–95.

20 Ciocca M. Medication and supplement use by athletes. *Clinics in Sports Medicine*. 2005; 24(3): 719–38.

21 Bahrke MS, Yesalis CE. Abuse of anabolic androgenic steroids and related substances in sport and exercise. *Current Opinion in Pharmacology*. 2004; 4(6): 614–20.

22 Hernandez-Nieto L, Bruguera M, Bombi J, Camacho L, Rozman C. Benign liver-cell adenoma associated with long-term administration of an androgenic-anabolic steroid (methandienone). *Cancer*. 1977; 40(4): 1761–4.

23 Stimac D, Milic S, Dintinjana RD, Kovac D, Ristic S. Androgenic/anabolic steroid-induced toxic hepatitis. *Journal of Clinical Gastroenterology*. 2002; 35(4): 350–2.

24 Socas L, Zumbado M, Pérez-Luzardo O, Ramos A, Pérez C, Hernández JR, Boada LD. Hepatocellular adenomas associated with anabolic androgenic steroid abuse in bodybuilders: a report of two cases and a review of the literature. *British Journal of Sports Medicine*. 2005; 39: e27.

25 Boyd PR, Mark GJ. Multiple hepatic adenomas and a hepatocellular carcinoma in a man on oral methyl testosterone for eleven years. *Cancer*. 1977; 40(4): 1765–70.

26 Hartgens F, Kuipers H, Wijnen JA, Keizer HA. Body composition, cardiovascular risk factors and liver function in long-term androgenic-anabolic steroids using bodybuilders three months after drug withdrawal. *International Journal of Sports Medicine*. 1996; 17(6): 429–33.

27 Gordon BS, Wolf J, Krause T, Shai F. Peliosis hepatis and cholestasis following administration of norethandrolone. *American Journal of Clinical Pathology*. 1960; 33: 156–65.

28 Cabasso A. Peliosis hepatis in a young adult bodybuilder. *Medicine and Science in Sports and Exercise*. 1994; 26(1): 2–4.

29 McGiven AR. Peliosis hepatis: case report and review of pathogenesis. *Journal of Pathology*. 1970; 101(3): 283–5.

30 Naeim F, Copper PH, Semion AA. Peliosis hepatis: possible etiologic role of anabolic steroids. *Archives of Pathology*. 1973; 95(4): 284–5.

31 Kuipers H, Wijnen JA, Hartgens F, Willems SM. Influence of anabolic steroids on body composition, blood pressure, lipid profile and liver functions in body builders. *International Journal of Sports Medicine*. 1991; 12(4): 413–18.

32 Lenders JW, Demacker PN, Vos JA, Jansen PL, Hoitsma AJ, van't Laar A, Thien T. Deleterious effects of anabolic steroids on serum lipoproteins, blood pressure, and liver function in amateur body builders. *International Journal of Sports Medicine.* 1988; 9(1): 19–23.

33 Melchert RB, Welder AA. Cardiovascular effects of androgenic-anabolic steroids. *Medicine and Science in Sports and Exercise.* 1995; 27(9): 1252–62.

34 Glazer G. Atherogenic effects of anabolic steroids on serum lipid levels: a literature review. *Archives of Internal Medicine.* 1991; 151(10): 1925–33.

35 Kantor MA, Bianchini A, Bernier D, Sady SP, Thompson PD. Androgens reduce HDL2-cholesterol and increase hepatic triglyceride lipase activity. *Medicine and Science in Sports and Exercise.* 1985; 17(4): 462–5.

36 Sullivan ML, Martinez CM, Gennis P, Gallagher EJ. The cardiac toxicity of anabolic steroids. *Progress in Cardiovascular Diseases.* 1998; 41(1): 1–15.

37 Ansell JE, Tiarks C, Fairchild VK. Coagulation abnormalities associated with the use of anabolic steroids. *American Heart Journal.* 1993; 125(2 Pt 1): 367–71.

38 Ferenchick GS. Anabolic/androgenic steroid abuse and thrombosis: is there a connection? *Medical Hypotheses.* 1999; 35(1): 27–31.

39 Dickerman RD, Schaller F, Prather I, McConathy WJ. Sudden cardiac death in a 20-year-old bodybuilder using anabolic steroids. *Cardiology.* 1995; 86(2): 172–3.

40 Ferenchick GS, Adelman S. Myocardial infarction associated with anabolic steroid use in a previously healthy 37-year-old weight lifter. *American Heart Journal.* 1992; 124(2): 507–8.

41 Frankle MA, Eichberg R, Zachariah SB. Anabolic androgenic steroids and a stroke in an athlete: case report. *Archives of Physical Medicine and Rehabilitation.* 1988; 69(8): 632–3.

42 Huie MJ. An acute myocardial infarction occurring in an anabolic steroid user. *Medicine and Science in Sports and Exercise.* 1994; 26(4): 408–13.

43 Kennedy MC, Lawrence C. Anabolic steroid abuse and cardiac death. *Medical Journal of Australia.* 1993; 158(5): 346–8.

44 Luke JL, Farb A, Virmani R, Sample RH. Sudden cardiac death during exercise in a weight lifter using anabolic androgenic steroids: pathological and toxicological findings. *Journal of Forensic Science.* 1990; 35(6): 1441–7.

45 McCarthy K, Tang AT, Dalrymple-Hay MJ, Haw MP. Ventricular thrombosis and systemic embolism in bodybuilders: etiology and management. *Annals of Thoracic Surgery.* 2000; 70(2): 658–60.

46 McNutt RA, Ferenchick GS, Kirlin PC, Hamlin NJ. Acute myocardial infarction in a 22-year-old world class weight lifter using anabolic steroids. *American Journal of Cardiology.* 1988; 62(1): 164.

47 Nieminen MS, Rämö MP, Viitasalo M, Heikkilä P, Karjalainen J, Mäntysaari M, Heikkilä J. Serious cardiovascular side effects of large doses of anabolic steroids in weight lifters. *European Heart Journal.* 1996; 17(10): 1576–83.

48 MacDougall JD, McKelvie RS, Moroz DE, Sale DG, McCartney N, Buick F. Factors affecting blood pressure during heavy weight lifting and static contractions. *Journal of Applied Physiology.* 1992; 73(4): 1590–7.

49 MacDougall JD, Tuxen D, Sale DG, Moroz JR, Sutton JR. Arterial blood pressure response to heavy resistance exercise. *Journal of Applied Physiology.* 1985; 58(3): 785–90.

50 Alaraj AM, Chamoun RB, Dahdaleh NS, Haddad GF, Comair YG. Spontaneous subdural haematoma in anabolic steroids dependent weight lifters: reports of two cases and review of literature. *Acta Neurochirurgica* (Vienna). 2005; 147(1): 85–7; discussion 7–8.

51 Urhausen A, Hölpes R, Kindermann W. One- and two- dimensional echocardiography in bodybuilders using anabolic steroids. *European Journal of Applied Physiology*. 1989; 58: 633–40.

52 Sachtleben TR, Berg KE, Elias BA, Cheatham JP, Felix GL, Hofschire PJ. The effects of anabolic steroids on myocardial structure and cardiovascular fitness. *Medicine and Science in Sports and Exercise*. 1993; 25(11): 1240–5.

53 D'Andrea A, Caso P, Salerno G, Scarafile R, De Corato G, Mita C, Di Salvo G, Severino S, Cuomo S, Liccardo B, Esposito N, Calabrò R. Left ventricular early myocardial dysfunction after chronic misuse of anabolic androgenic steroids: a Doppler myocardial and strain imaging analysis. *British Journal of Sports Medicine*. 2007; 41(3): 149–55.

54 Ferenchick GS. Association of steroid use with cardiomyopathy in athletes. *American Journal of Medicine*. 1991; 91: 562.

55 Herschman Z. Cardiac effects of anabolic steroids. *Anesthesiology*. 1990; 72(4): 772–3.

56 Menkis AH, Daniel JK, McKenzie FN, Novick RJ, Kostuk WJ, Pflugfelder PW. Cardiac transplantation after myocardial infarction in a 24-year-old bodybuilder using anabolic steroids. *Clinical Journal of Sport Medicine*. 1991; 1(2): 138–40.

57 Gruber AJ, Pope HG Jr. Psychiatric and medical effects of anabolic-androgenic steroid use in women. *Psychotherapy and Psychosomatics*. 2000; 69(1): 19–26.

58 Parrott AC, Choi PY, Davies M. Anabolic steroid use by amateur athletes: effects upon psychological mood states. *Journal of Sports Medicine and Physical Fitness*. 1994; 34(3): 292–8.

59 Pope HG Jr, Kouri EM, Hudson JI. Effects of supraphysiologic doses of testosterone on mood and aggression in normal men: a randomized controlled trial. *Archives of General Psychiatry*. 2000; 57(2): 133–40; discussion 55–6.

60 Porcerelli JH, Sandler BA. Anabolic-androgenic steroid abuse and psychopathology. *Psychiatric Clinics of North America*. 1998; 21(4): 829–33.

61 Su TP, Pagliaro M, Schmidt PJ, Pickar D, Wolkowitz O, Rubinow R. Neuropsychiatric effects of anabolic steroids in male normal volunteers. *Journal of the American Medical Association*. 1993; 269(21): 2760–4.

62 Tricker R, Casaburi R, Storer TW, Clevenger B, Berman N, Shirazi A, Bhasin S. The effects of supraphysiological doses of testosterone on angry behavior in healthy eugonadal men: a clinical research center study. *Journal of Clinical Endocrinology and Metabolism*. 1996; 81(10): 3754–8.

63 Conacher GN, Workman DG. Violent crime possibly associated with anabolic steroid use. *American Journal of Psychiatry*. 1989; 146(5): 679.

64 Pope HG Jr, Katz DL. Homicide and near-homicide by anabolic steroid users. *Journal of Clinical Psychiatry*. 1990; 51(1): 28–31.

65 Choi PY, Pope HG Jr. Violence toward women and illicit androgenic-anabolic steroid use. *Annals of Clinical Psychiatry*. 1994; 6(1): 21–5.

66 Thiblin I, Lindquist O, Rajs J. Cause and manner of death among users of anabolic androgenic steroids. *Journal of Forensic Science*. 2000; 45(1): 16–23.

67 Thiblin I, Runeson B, Rajs J. Anabolic androgenic steroids and suicide. *Annals of Clinical Psychiatry*. 1999; 11(4): 223–31.

68 Allnutt S, Chaimowitz G. Anabolic steroid withdrawal depression: a case report [letter]. *Canadian Journal of Psychiatry*. 1994; 39: 317–18.

69 Brower KJ, Blow FC, Beresford TP, Fuelling C. Anabolic-androgenic steroid dependence. *Journal of Clinical Psychiatry*. 1989; 50(1): 31–3.

70 Tennant F, Black DL, Voy RO. Anabolic steroid dependence with opioid-type features. *New England Journal of Medicine*. 1988; 319(9): 578.

71 Brower KJ, Blow FC, Young JP, Hill EM. Symptoms and correlates of anabolic-androgenic steroid dependence. *British Journal of Addiction*. 1991; 86(6): 759–68.

72 Kashkin KB, Kleber HD. Hooked on hormones? An anabolic steroid addiction hypothesis. *Journal of the American Medical Association*. 1989; 262(22): 3166–70.

73 Kanayama G, Cohane GH, Weiss RD, Pope HG. Past anabolic-androgenic steroid use among men admitted for substance abuse treatment: an underrecognized problem? *Journal of Clinical Psychiatry*. 2003; 64(2): 156–60.

74 Giannini AJ, Miller N, Kocjan DK. Treating steroid abuse: a psychiatric perspective. *Clinical Pediatrics*. 1991; 30: 538–42.

75 Király CL, Alén M, Rahkila P, Horsmanheimo M. Effect of androgenic-anabolic steroids on the sebaceous gland in power athletes. *Acta Dermato-Venereologica*. 1987; 67(1): 36–40.

76 Dohle GR, Smit M, Weber RF. Androgens and male fertility. *World Journal of Urology*. 2003; 21: 341–5.

77 Boyadjiev NP, Georgieva RJ, Massaldjieva RI, Gueorguiev SI. Reversible hypogonadism and azoospermia as a result of anabolic-androgenic steroid use in a body builder with personality disorder: a case report. *Journal of Sports Medicine and Physical Fitness*. 2000; 40: 271–4.

78 Wemyss-Holden SA, Hamdy FC, Hastie KJ. Steroid abuse in athletes, prostatic enlargement and bladder outflow obstruction: is there a relationship? *British Journal of Urology*. 1994; 74(4): 476–8.

79 Parssinen M, Seppala T. Steroid use and long-term health risks in former athletes. *Sports Medicine*. 2002; 32(2): 83–94.

80 Battista V, Combs J, Warme WJ. Asynchronous bilateral achilles tendon ruptures and androstenediol use. *American Journal of Sports Medicine*. 2003; 31(6): 1007–9.

81 Michna H. Tendon injuries induced by exercise and anabolic steroids in experimental mice. *International Orthopaedics*. 1987; 11(2): 157–62.

82 Shahidi NT. A review of the chemistry, biological action, and clinical applications of anabolic-androgenic steroids. *Clinical Therapeutics*. 2001; 23(9): 1355–90.

83 Rich JD, Dickinson BP, Feller A, Pugatch D, Mylonakis E. The infectious complications of anabolic-androgenic steroid injection. *International Journal of Sports Medicine*. 1999; 20(8): 563–6.

84 Melia P, Pipe A, Greenberg L. The use of anabolic-androgenic steroids by Canadian students. *Clinical Journal of Sport Medicine*. 1996; 6(1): 9–14.

85 Birkeland K, Stray-Gundersen J, Hemmersbach P, Hallen J, Haug E, Bahr R. Effect of rhEPO administration on serum levels of sTfR and cycling performance. *Medicine and Science in Sports and Exercise*. 1999; 32(7): 1238–43.

86 Eichner ER. Better dead than second. *Journal of Laboratory and Clinical Medicine*. 1992; 120: 359–60.

87 Fotheringham W. Inquiry into Belgian cyclists' deaths raises new fears over EPO. *Guardian* (London) 2004 16 February.

88 Voet W. *Breaking the chain: drugs and cycling: the true story.* London: Yellow Jersey (Random House).

89 Lage J, Panizo C, Masdeu J, Rocha E. Cyclist's doping associated with cerebral sinus thrombosis. *Neurology.* 2002; 58: 665.

90 Lippi G, Franchini M, Salvagno G, Guidi G. Biochemistry, physiology, and complications of blood doping: facts and speculation. *Critical Reviews in Clinical Laboratory Sciences.* 2006; 43(4): 349–91.

91 Bennett C, Luminari S, Nissenson AR, Tallman MS, Klinge SA, McWilliams N, McKoy JM, Kim B, Lyons EA, Trifilio SM, Raisch DW, Evens AM, Kuzel TM, Schumock GT, Belknap SM, Locatelli F, Rossert J, Casadevall N. Pure red-call aplasia and epoietin therapy. *New England Journal of Medicine.* 2004; 351: 1403–8.

92 Yasuda J, Fujita Y, Matsuo T, Koinuma S, Hara S, Tazaki A, Onozaki M, Hashimoto M, Musha T, Ogawa K, Fujita H, Nakamura Y, Shiozaki H, Utsumi H. Erythropoietin regulates tumour growth of human malignancies. *Carcinogenesis.* 2003; 24: 1021–9.

93 Scheen A. Pharma-clinics: doping with erythropoietin or the misuse of therapeutic advances. *Revue Médicale de Liège.* 1998; 53(8): 499–502.

94 Shaskey DJ, Green GA. Sports hematology. *Sports Medicine.* 2000; 29(1): 27–38.

95 Dean H. Does exogenous growth hormone improve athletic performance? *Clinical Journal of Sport Medicine.* 2002; 12(4): 250–3.

96 Rennie MJ. Claims for the anabolic effects of growth hormone: a case of the Emperor's new clothes? *British Journal of Sports Medicine.* 2003; 37: 100–5.

97 Healy ML, Gibney J, Russell-Jones DL, Pentecost C, Croos P, Sönksen PH, Umpleby AM. High dose growth hormone exerts an anabolic effect at rest and during exercise in endurance-trained athletes. *Journal of Clinical Endocrinology and Metabolism.* 2003; 88: 5221–6.

98 Saugy M, Robinson N, Saudan C, Baume N, Avois L, Mangin P. Human growth hormone doping in sport. *British Journal of Sports Medicine.* 2006; 40(Suppl. I): i35–i9.

99 Jenkins P. Growth hormone and exercise: physiology, use and abuse. *Growth Hormone and IGF Research.* 2001; 11(Suppl. A): s71–s7.

100 Handlesman D. The rationale for banning human chorionic gonadotrophin and estrogen blockers in sport. *Journal of Clinical Endocrinology and Metabolism.* 2006; 91(5): 1646–53.

101 Thorsson A, Christiansen P, Ritzen M. Efficacy and safety of hormonal treatment of cryptorchisism: current state of the art. *Acta Paediatrica.* 2007; 96: 628–30.

102 Hutson J. Treatment of undescended testes: time for a change in European traditions. *Acta Paediatrica.* 2007; 96: 608–10.

103 Karila T, Hovatta O, Seppala T. Concomitant abuse of anaboloic androgenic steroids and human chorionic gonadotrophin impairs spermatogenesis in power athletes. *International Journal of Sports Medicine.* 2004; 25(4): 257–63.

104 Dawson RT, Harrison MW. Use of insulin as an anabolic agent. *British Journal of Sports Medicine.* 1997; 31: 259.

105 Reverter J, Tural C, Rosell A, Dominguez M, Sonmarti A. Self-induced insulin hypoglycemia in a bodybuilder. *Archives of Internal Medicine.* 1994; 154(2): 225–6.

106 Elkin SL, Brady S, Williams IP. Bodybuilders find it easy to obtain insulin to help them in training. *British Medical Journal*. 1997; 314: 1280.

107 Rich JD, Dickinson BP, Merriman NA, Thule PM. Insulin use by bodybuilders. *Journal of the American Medical Association*. 1998; 279(20): 1613.

108 Schoene RB, Giboney K, Schimmel C, Hagen J, Robinson J, Schoene RB, Sato W, Sullivan KN. Spirometry and airway reactivity in elite track and field athletes. *Clinical Journal of Sport Medicine*. 1997; 7(4): 257–61.

109 Ng'ang'a LW, Odhiambo JA, Mungai MW, Gicheha CM, Nderitu P, Maingi B, Macklem PT, Becklake MR. Prevalence of exercise-induced bronchospasm in Kenyan school children: an urban-rural comparison. *Thorax*. 1998; 53(11): 919–26.

110 Wilbur RL, Rundell KW, Szmedra L, Jenkinson D, Im J, Drake SD. Incidence of exercise-induced bronchoconstriction in Olympic winter sport athletes. *Medicine and Science in Sports and Exercise*. 2000; 32(4): 732–7.

111 Weiler JM, Ryan EJ. Asthma in US Olympic athletes who participated in the 1998 Winter Olympic Games. *Journal of Allergy and Clinical Immunology*. 2000; 106(2): 267–71.

112 Parsons JP, Mastronarda JG. Exercise-induced bronchoconstriction in athletes. *Chest*. 2005; 128(6): 3966–74.

113 Knopfl BH, Zeitoun LM, von Duvillard SP, Burki A, Bachlechner C, Kellar H. High incidence of exercise-induced bronchoconstriction in triathletes of the Swiss national team. *British Journal of Sports Medicine*. 2007; 41(8): 486–91.

114 Parsons JP, Kaeding C, Phillips G, Jarjoura D, Wadley G, Mastronarde JG. Prevalence of exercise-induced bronchospasm in a cohort of varsity college athletes. *Medicine and Science in Sports and Exercise*. 2007; 39(9): 1487–92.

115 Nelson HS. Is there a problem with inhaled long-acting beta-adrenergic agents? *Journal of Allergy and Clinical Immunology*. 2006; 117(1): 3–16.

116 Kelly HW. Risk versus benefit considerations for the beta-2-agonists. *Pharmacotherapy*. 2006; 26(9): 164S–174S.

117 Salpeter SR, Ormiston TM, Salpeter EE. Cardiovascular effects of beta-agonists in patients with asthma and COPD: a meta-analysis. *Chest*. 2004; 125(6): 2309–21.

118 Walters EH, Gibson PG, Lasserson TJ, Walters JA. Long-acting beta2-agonists for chronic asthma in adults and children where background therapy contains varied or no inhaled corticosteroid. *Cochrane Database of Systematic Reviews*. 2003; Issue 4. Art. No.: CD001385. DOI: 10.1002/14651858.CD001385.pub2.

119 ZuWallack R, Adelglass J, Clifford DP, Duke SP, Wire PD, Faris M, Harding SM. Long-term efficacy and safety of fluticasone propionate powder administered once or twice daily via inhaler to patients with moderate asthma. *Chest*. 2000; 118(2): 303–12.

120 Sizonenko PC. Effects of inhaled or nasal glucocorticosteroids on adrenal function and growth. *Journal of Pediatric Endocrinology and Medicine*. 2002; 15(1): 5–26.

121 Claremont AD, Costill DL, Fink W, Van Handel P. Heat tolerance following diuretic induced dehydration. *Medicine and Science in Sports and Exercise*. 1976; 8(4): 239–43.

122 Caldwell JE, Ahonen E, Nousianen U. Differential effects of sauna-, diuretic-, and exercise-induced dehydration. *Journal of Applied Physiology*. 1984; 57(4): 1018–23.

123   Armstrong LE, Costill DL, Fink WJ. Influence of diuretic-induced dehydration on competitive running performance. *Medicine and Science in Sports and Exercise*. 1985; 17(4): 456–61.

124   Watson G, Judelson DA, Armstrong LE, Yeargin SW, Case DJ, Manesh CM. Influence of diuretic induced dehydration on competitive sprint and power performance. *Medicine and Science in Sports and Exercise*. 2005; 37(7): 1168–74.

125   Laties VG, Weiss B. The amphetamine margin in sports. *Federation Proceedings*. 1981; 40(12): 2689–92.

126   Lippi G, Franchini M, Guidi GC. Switch off the light on cycling, switch off the light on doping. *British Journal of Sports Medicine*. 1987 November 5 [e-pub ahead of print].

127   Jacobs W. Fatal amphetamine associated cardiotoxicity and its medicolegal implications. *American Journal of Forensic Medicine and Pathology*. 2006; 27(2): 156–60.

128   Degenhardt L, Copeland J, Dillon P. Recent trends in the use of "club drugs": an Australian review. *Substance Use and Misuse*. 2005; 40(9–10): 1241–56.

129   Green AR, Cross AJ, Goodwin GM. Review of the pharmacology and clinical pharmacology of 3,4-methylenedioxymethamphetamine (MDMA or Ecstasy). *Psychopharmacology* (Berlin). 1995; 119(3): 247–60.

130   Karlsen SN, Spigset O, Slordal L. The dark side of ecstasy: neuropsychiatric symptoms after exposure to 3,4-methylenedioxymethamphetamine. *Basic and Clinical Pharmacology and Toxicology*. 2007 November 28 [e-pub ahead of print]).

131   Hall AP, Henry JA. Acute toxic effects of "Ecstasy" (MDMA) and related compounds: overview of pathophysiology and clinical management. *British Journal of Anaesthesia*. 2006; 96(6): 678–85.

132   Gruber AJ, Pope HG Jr. Ephedrine use among 36 female weight lifters. *American Journal on Addictions*. 1998; 7(4): 256–61.

133   Centers for Disease Control and Prevention (CDC). Adverse events associated with ephedrine containing products – Texas, December 1993 – September, 1995. MMWR *Morbidity and Mortality Weekly Report*. 1996; 45(37): 689–93.

134   Cupp MJ. Herbal remedies: adverse effects and drug interactions. *American Family Physician*. 1999; 59(5): 1239–45.

135   Haller CA, Benowitz NL. Adverse cardiovascular and central nervous system events associated with dietary supplements containing ephedra alkaloids. *New England Journal of Medicine*. 2000; 343(25): 1833–8.

136   Izzo A, Ernst E. Interactions between herbal medications and prescribed drugs: a systematic review. *Drugs*. 2001; 61(15): 2163–75.

137   Semenuk D, Link MS, Homoud MK, Contreras R, Theoharides TC, Wang PJ, Estes NA III. Adverse cardiovascular events associated with ma huang, a herbal source of ephedrine. *Mayo Clinic Proceedings*. 2002; 77(1): 12–16.

138   Shekelle P, Hardy ML, Morton SC, Maglione M, Mojica WA, Suttorp MJ, Rhodes, SL, Jungvig L, Gagné J. Efficacy and safety of ephedra and ephedrine for weight loss and athletic performance: a meta-analysis. *Journal of the American Medical Association*. 2003; 289(12): 1537–45.

139   Andrews R, Charla P, Brown DL. Cardiovascular effects of ephedra alkaloids: a comprehensive review. *Progress in Cardiovascular Diseases*. 2005; 47(4): 217–25.

140   Pittler MH, Schmidt K, Ernst E. Adverse events of herbal food supplements for body weight reduction: systematic review. *Obesity Reviews*. 2005; 6(2): 93–111.

141 Avois L, Robinson N, Saudan C, Baume N, Mangin P, Saugy M. Central nervous system stimulants and sport practice. *British Journal of Sports Medicine*. 2006; 40(Suppl. 1): i16–i20.

142 Weider AA, Melchert RB. Cardiotoxic effects of cocaine and anabolic-androgenic steroids in the athlete. *Journal of Pharmacological and Toxicological Methods*. 1993; 29(2): 61–8.

143 Frishman WH, DelVecchio A, Sanai S, Ismail A. Cardiovascular manifestations of substance abuse part 1: Cocaine. *Heart Disease*. 2003; 5(3): 187–201.

144 Egred M, Davis GK. Cocaine and the heart. *Postgraduate Medical Journal*. 2005; 81(959): 568–71.

145 Aforso L, Mohammad T, Thatai D. Crack whips the heart: a review of the cardiotoxicity of cocaine. *American Journal of Cardiology*. 2007; 100(6): 1040–3.

146 Glauser J, Queen JB. An overview of non-cardiac cocaine toxicity. *Journal of Emergency Medicine*. 2007; 32(2): 181–6.

147 Restrepro CS, Carrilla JA, Martinez S, Ojeda P, Rivera AL, Hatta A. Pulmonary complications from cocaine and cocaine-based substances: imaging manifestations. *Radiographics*. 2007; 27(4): 941–56.

148 Mnadi CU, Mimiko OA, McCurtis HL, Cadet JL. Neuropsychiatric effects of cocaine use disorders. *Journal of the National Medical Association*. 2005; 97(11): 1504–15.

149 Slatkoff J, Greenfield B. Pharmacologic treatment of attention deficit/hyperactivity disorder in adults. *Expert Opinion on Investigational Drugs*. 2006; 15(6): 649–67.

150 King S, Griffin S, Hodges Z, Weatherly H, Asseburg C, Richardson G, Golder S, Taylor E, Drummond M, Riemsma R. A systematic review and economic model of the effectiveness and cost-effectiveness of methylphenidate, dexamfetamine and atomoxetine for the treatment of attention deficit hyperactivity disorder in children and adolescents. *Health Technology Assessment*. 2006; 10(23): iii–iv, xiii-146.

151 Nicholson B. Responsible prescribing of opioids for the management of chronic pain. *Drugs*. 2003; 63(1): 17–32.

152 Kalant H. Adverse effects of cannabis on health: an update of the literature since *Progress in Neuro-Psychopharmacology and Biological Psychiatry*. 2004; 28(5): 849–63.

153 Macleod J, Oakes R, Copello A, Crome I, Egger M, Hickman M, Oppenkuwski T, Stokes-Lampard H, Daverg Smith G. Psychological and social sequelae of cannabis and other illicit drug use by young people: a systematic review of longitudinal, general population studies. *Lancet*. 2004; 363(9421): 1579–88.

154 Hall WD. Cannnabis use and the mental health of young people. *Australian and New Zealand Journal of Psychiatry*. 2006; 40(2): 105–13.

155 Tetrault JM, Crothers K, Moore BA, Mehra R, Concato J, Fiellin DA. Effects of marijuana smoking on pulmonary function and respiratory complications: a systematic review. *Archives of Internal Medicine*. 2007; 167(3): 221–8.

156 Aldington S, Williams M, Nowitz M, Weatherall M, Pritchard A, McNaughton A, Robinson G, Beasley R. Effects of cannabis on pulmonary structures, function and symptoms. *Thorax*. 2007; 62(12): 1058–63.

157 Nicholas W. Complications associated with the use of corticosteroids in the treatment of athletic injuries. *Clinical Journal of Sport Medicine*. 2005; 15(5): 370–5.

158 Dvorak J, Feddermann N, Grimm K. Glucocorticosteroids in football: use and misuse. *British Journal of Sports Medicine*. 2006; 40(Suppl. 1): i48–i54.

159 Keenan G. Management of complications of glucocorticoid therapy. *Clinics in Chest Medicine.* 1997; 18: 507–20.

160 Hengge UR, Ruzicka T, Schwartz RD. Adverse effects of topical glucocorticosteroids. *Journal of the American Academy of Dermatology.* 2006; 54(1): 1–15.

161 Williams LC, Nesbitt LT. Update on systemic glucocorticosteroids in dermatology. *Dermatologic Clinics.* 2001; 19(1): 63–77.

162 Warrington TP, Bostwick JM. Psychiatric adverse effects of glucocorticosteroids. *Mayo Clinic Proceedings.* 2006; 81(10): 1361–7.

163 Mazziotti G, Angeli A, Bilezikian JP, Canalis E, Giustina A. Glucocorticoid-induced osteoporosis: an update. *Trends in Endocrinology and Metabolism.* 2006; 17(4): 144–9.

164 Riebe D, Maresh CM, Armstrong LE, Kenefick RW, Castelloni JW, Echegaray ME, Clark BA, Camaione DN. Effects of oral and intravenous rehydration on ratings of perceived exertion and thirst. *Medicine and Science in Sports and Medicine.* 1997; 29(1): 117–24.

165 Keneflick RW, O'Moore KM, Mahood NV, Castellani JW. Rapid IV versus oral rehydration: responses to subsequent heat stress. *Medicine and Science in Sports and Medicine.* 2006; 38(12): 2125–31.

14 Conclusions

Jean L Fourcroy

The United States Anti-Doping Agency (USADA) is committed to provide a testing program that achieves both deterrence and detection; it was designed with athlete concerns in mind. USADA's research program contributes significantly to the worldwide anti-doping effort. In addition, USADA offers a broad-based education program that provides a forum for clean sport at all levels, emphasizing the ideals of the Olympic movement.[1] None of this would be possible without the vision and integrity of dedicated scientists around the world, without which we would not have the protection for our clean athletes to engage in fair competition. Through our enthusiasm, innovation, ingenuity, transparency, and communication, USADA exemplifies the quality of anti-doping agencies worldwide.[2,3]

Doping is defined as the administration of, or use by competing athletes of, any substances foreign to the body or of any physiological substance taken in abnormal quantity or taken by an abnormal route of entry into the body with the sole intention of increasing in an artificial and unfair manner his or her performance in competition. Performance enhancement includes recovery, improved focus, concentration, and alteration of the perception of fatigue. We know that doping is unfair and unethical and should be banned from competitions. Doping and performance enhancement is not limited to elite sports but appears to command our everyday life at all ages.[4-7]

Athletes of all ages have discovered many approaches to improve performance, focus and recovery. Many of the products used for doping or enhancement were new and novel in the twentieth century. Some, like androstenedione, were until recently dietary supplements, finally removed from the market by the combined efforts of USADA and the Coalition for Anabolic Steroid Precursor and Ephedra Regulation (CASPER) group supporting the Sweeney–Osborne Bill.[8,9]

In previous chapters, science's best have shared their expertise to protect our athletes. Above all, the health of our athletes comes first, and this discussion is also included. The most important event is the testing ability demonstrated by our elite laboratories around the world. Of course, none of this would be possible without the validation and accreditation of laboratories approved by the highest standards.[2,3] Several chapters have pointed out these standards.[3,10,11] The importance of a process to identify new analyses is part of this excellence.[11–13]

1 Androgens and anabolic steroids (AAS)

Androgens came on the scene relatively recently with the first identification and development of new androgenic drug products in the 1930s.[13–18] Athletes quickly became aware of their anabolic promise, partly through such publications as the *Underground Steroid Handbook.*[19] The mass production and use of these AAS have grown, including use of dietary supplements such as androstenedione, a potent androgen, familiar to both baseball players and the German Democratic Republic government.[14,20–22] Prior to a 1962 review of drugs approved by the Food and Drug Administration, many ineffective and even unstudied combination products were available.[23]

It is important to remember that most of this AAS development occurred before 1962, when effectiveness of the drug was not an issue. The Food and Drug Administration (FDA) website is an important source for both the FDA historical background and past and current legislation.[24] A myriad of AAS drugs were marketed for a variety of unproven conditions, including, prepubertal cryptorchidism, evidence of hypogonadism, and male senescence. A variety of claims in advertisements suggested that both their anabolic and their catabolic effects retard tissue depletion, speed tissue building and act as an anabolic stimulant.[25] It did not take long for athletes to abuse these compounds for their anabolic effects.[19]

USADA took the lead in initiating legislation to protect the health of both athletes and the public. The Anabolic Steroid Control Act of 2004 stipulated a ban on over-the-counter steroid precursors, increased penalties for making, selling or possessing illegal steroid precursors, and funds for the preventive education of children. The passage of this Act was due to the efforts of CASPER, with representatives from leading medical associations and public health and sports organizations.[8] As a result of this Act, most androgenic dietary supplements, with the exception of dehydroepiandrosterone (DHEA), were removed from the market. Almost every day, however, a new website advertises another designer steroid, or presumed steroid, to the public.[26] Providers and athletes of all ages must be aware that these designer steroids are unproven and in some cases unsafe.

The attempt to mask a new compound to escape detection is the essence of the tetrahydrogestrinone (THG) story, THG being a designer molecule was developed and used illicitly to improve athletic performance. Although its structure is closely related to gestrinone, a 19-norprogestin, and resembles that of trenbolone, it did not appear ever to have been marketed previously (see Chapters 5, 12 and 13).

Identifying and profiling steroids is not a challenge for good scientists. Two tests helped laboratories identify the possibility of AAS use. These include the testosterone to epitestosterone ratio (T:E) and the carbon isotope ratio

(CIR). These tests provided an important step in the validation of anabolic steroid doping.[10,27–30] The chapter on CIR was in fact written by one of the developers of this test. Both CIR and testosterone to epitesoterone ratio tests represented important steps in testing.

The recognition of isotopes has become an important part of testing even outside the doping world. To define an isotope, it is important to know that the atomic mass of an atom is defined by the weight of the number of protons and neutrons in the nucleus. This technology will be important in many other areas of clinical research.[31]

2 Blood doping

How many ways can an athlete improve oxygen carrying capacity? He or she can increase the number of red blood cells, add blood or try erythropoietin (EPO). Red blood cells perform the essential function of transporting oxygen throughout the body. Chapter 9 gives us a clear understanding of the effect of erythrocyte volume on human athletic performance.[32] Erythropoietin acts as a blood production stimulant, while androgens and anabolic steroids also increase the production of red blood cells.

Blood doping is an alternative method of increasing the number of red blood cells in an attempt to improve athletic performance. In the past, this was accomplished by transfusion, either stored or donated. It enables performance improvements in endurance sports because of the extra oxygen carrying capacity. The practice has been outlawed, not just because it is unfair but because of the dangers involved.[32–34]

The pharmaceutical development of a recombinant EPO provided a new challenge. This drug is the same as the body's natural erythropoietin, a glycoprotein produced by the kidneys that circulates through the bloodstream to bone marrow, where it stimulates red blood cell production. Athletes quickly caught on to the enhancement possibilities of this new, chemical version of EPO. Important methods of detection have been described in this book.[35–41]

3 Growth hormones

Growth hormone (GH) is thought to have been first abused prior to 1985 using extracted pituitary hormones. Cadaver GH was approved for treatment of growth hormone deficiency diseases as early as the 1960s. However, in the 1980s, researchers discovered that Creutzfeldt–Jakob disease (CJD) could be transmitted from cadavers to cadaver GH users, and its use was discontinued in most countries. Today, recombinant GH is made in unlimited, though expensive, quantities, with several major distributors worldwide. Growth hormones remain an important enhancement tool for athletes.

The safety issues related to GH abuse are well understood since it mimics the disease of hypersecretion; that is, acromegaly. Long-term administration of high doses of GH is potentially dangerous. The misuse of GH has increased dramatically as a result of its increased recombinant availability and, until recently, the lack of a test to detect its use.

There is a complicated regulation of growth hormones and the metabolic pathway or pharmacodynamics markers which will probably allow for "indirect detection" of exogenous growth hormones.[42] The most useful markers of GH abuse include the variation between the 22-kD and 20-kD GH isomers as well as metabolic markers of GH including insulin-like growth factor I, acid-labile subunit, IFG-I binding protein 3, IGF-I binding protein 2, osteocalcin, C-terminal propetide of Type I procollagen, procollagen Type III, Type I collagen telopeptide. Tests have been calibrated for "elite" athletes using a large amount of post-competition data with adjustments for age.[43–48]

Dr Sönksen has been an important leader at the Olympic level in the recognition and development of growth horme tests; his chapter shares some of that history. A devastating skiing accident left him with a spinal cord injury but we are fortunate that this has not slowed him down.

4 Gene doping

WADA was ahead of the game when it first put together a meeting to discuss the issues of gene doping.[49] Dr Friedmann, who has been a leader in the therapeutic use of genes, has given us an excellent summary of the history.[49] Early disease targets for gene therapy tended to be inborn errors of metabolism. In principle, all one had to do was to put the gene into the right cell at the right time to replace a broken or missing gene. It is fair to ask where genes will take us for the medicine of the future.[50–53]

5 The healthy athlete

The most important issue in this book concerns the health of our athletes and the ethics of these challenges. We always benefit from the words of Dr Pipe, who has been an important scientist in this area.[54–56] When faced with issues of doping and sports in the 1980s, Canada was determined to understand the prevalence of this problem at all ages. This chapter on the healthy athlete carefully points out what we know about the health risks of doping – and there are many. Every physician should be aware of these risks for both male and female athletes. The female athlete triad is a combination of three interrelated conditions that are associated with athletic training: disordered eating, amenorrhea and osteoporosis.[57,58] The performance-enhancing drugs most often abused by students are anabolic steroids. A recent report from the government reminds us of the prevalence of this problem in our community.[59,60]

6 The ethics of biomedical enhancement

The ethics of biomedical enhancement or the use of drugs in sports is an ongoing dialog with the Hastings Center and Dr T. Murray. There are many ethical issues raised in any doping research protocols. At the first USADA summit in October 2000, we agreed that ethics should be part of every question on sports and doping. These questions are just as important to keep in mind today. Dr Murray points out in a recent article that

> the spirit of sport is in fact the celebration of the human spirit, body and mind, and is characterized by the following values: ethics, fair play and honesty, health, excellence in performance, character and education. Equally important is fun, joy and teamwork, dedication and commitment, respect for rules and laws, respect for self and other participants, courage, community and solidarity.[61]

We can all agree with these high ideals.

7 Summary

I have been blessed to be a part of this unique scientific community, but we are all indebted to the many heroes who advanced the science that contributed to this book. It is clear that many extraordinary individuals set the stage for the high level of science we see today in the WADA-accredited laboratories. Of particular note is Dr Manfred Donike, an international cyclist, who identified the importance of testing and the quality of the science. He set many early standards including the Cologne workshops, which shared important scientific knowledge.[62-64]

I speak on behalf of the Board and dedicated staff of USADA when I say that our commitment to science and the health of our athletes is very strong and of great importance.

8 References

1 United States Anti-Doping Agency [homepage on the internet]. Available from www.usantidoping.org (accessed February 4, 2008).
2 Bowers LD Ensuring quality results in a global testing system. This book, Chapter 2.
3 WADA International Standard for Laboratories, version 5. Available from http://www.wadaama.org/rtecontent/document/lab_aug_04.pdf (accessed December 16, 2007).
4 The George Mitchell Report. Available from http://mlb.mlb.com/mlb/news/mitchell/index.jsp; http://files.mlb.com/summary.pdf (accessed February 4, 2008).
5 The Taylor Hooton Foundation. Fighting steroid abuse. Available from http://www.taylorhooton.org/ (accessed February 4, 2008).
6 Kuehn BM. Many teens abusing medications. *Journal of the American Medical Association*. 2007; 297(6): 578–80.
7 National Institute on Drug Abuse (NIDA). NIDA initiative targets increasing teen use of anabolic steroids. Available from http://www.nida.nih.gov/ NIDA_notes/NNvol15N3/Initiative.html (accessed February 4, 2008).

8 Coalition for Anabolic Steroid Precursor and Ephedra Regulation (CASPER). Sweeney-Osborne introduce bill aimed at curbing steroid precursors. Available from http://www.casper207.com/files/PROctober92002.pdf (accessed February 4, 2008).

9 Senate Bill. 2195 [108th]: Anabolic Steroid Control Act of 2004. Available from http://www.govtrack.us/congress/bill.xpd?bill=s108-2195 (accessed February 4, 2008).

10 Aguilera R. Isotope ratio mass spectroscopy: carbon isotope ratio analysis. This book, Chapter 6.

11 Ayotte C. Testing for anabolic agents. This book, Chapter 4.

12 Death AK, McGrath KC, Kazlauskas R, Handelsman DJ. Tetrahydrogestrinone is a potent androgen and progestin. *Journal of Critical Endocrinology and Metabolism.* 2004; 89: 2498–500.

13 Jasuja R, Catlin DH, Miller A, Chang YC, Herbst KL, Starcevic B, Artaza JN, Singh R, Datta G, Sarkissian A, Chandsawangbhuwana C, Baker M, Bhasin S. Tetrahydrogestrinone is an androgenic steroid that stimulates androgen receptor-mediated, myogenic differentiation in C3H10T1/2 multipotent mesenchymal cells and promotes muscle accretion in orchidectomized male rats. *Endocrinology.* 2005; 146: 4472–8.

14 Clark R. Anabolic androgenic steroids: historical background, physiology, typical use and side effects. This book, Chapter 3.

15 Fourcroy, J. Designer steroids: past, present and future. *Current Opinion in Endocrinology and Diabetes.* 2000; 13(3): 306–9.

16 Hoberman JM, Yesalis CE. The history of synthetic testosterone. *Scientific American.* 1995; 272: 76–81.

17 Kochakian CD. The evolution from "the male hormone" to anabolic-androgenic steroids. *Alabama Journal of Medical Sciences.* 1988; 25: 96–102.

18 Kochakian CD. How it was: anabolic action of steroids and remembrances. Birmingham: University of Alabama School of Medicine, 1984.

19 Duchaine D. American steroids both oral and injectable. In: *Underground steroid handbook (II) update.* Marina Del Rey, CA: Power Distributors;

20 Dickman S. East Germany: science in the diservice of the state. *Science.* 1991; 254: 24–7.

21 Franke WW, Berendonk B. Hormonal doping and androgenization of athletes: a secret program of the German Democratic Republic government. *Clinical Chemistry.* 1997; 43(7): 1262–79.

22 Androstenedione. Definitions from http://en.wikipedia.org/wiki/Androstenedione (accessed February 4, 2008).

23 FDA History website. The Kefauver-Harris drug amendments are passed, October 10, 1962. Available from http://www.fda.gov/centennial/this_week/41_oct_08_oct_014.html (accessed February 4, 2008).

24 FDA [homepage on the internet]. Available from http://www.FDA.gov (accessed February 4, 2008).

25 Advertisement. *New England Journal of Medicine* advertising section xvii. 1962; April 12.

26 How to obtain anabolic steroids. Available from http://www.legalsteroids.com (accessed February 4, 2008).

27 Aguilera R, Chapman TE, Starcevic B, Hatton CK, Catlin DH. Performance characteristics of a carbon isotope ratio method for detecting doping with testosterone

based on urine diols: controls and athletes with elevated testosterone/epitestosterone ratios. *Clinical Chemistry*. 2001; 47(2): 292–300.

28 Catlin DH, Cowan DA, de la Torre R, Donike M, Fraisse D, Oftebro H, Hatton CK, Starcevic B, Becchi M, de la Torre X, Norli H, Geyer H, Walker CJ. Urinary testosterone (T) to epitestosterone (E) ratios by GC/MS. I. Initial comparison of uncorrected T/E in six international laboratories. *Journal of Mass Spectrometry*. 1996; 31: 297–402.

29 Donike M, Rauth S. Evaluation of longitudinal studies, the determination of subject based reference ranges of the testosterone/epitestosterone ratio. In: Donike M, Geyer H. Gotzmann A, Mareck-Engelke U, Rauth S. eds. *Proceedings of the Eleventh Cologne Workshop on Dope Analysis, March 7–12, 1993*. Cologne: Sport und Buch Strauβ, 1994; 33–9.

30 Shackleton CH, Phillips A, Chang T, Li Y. Confirming testosterone administration by isotope ratio mass spectrometric analysis of urinary androstanediols. *Steroids*. 1997; 62: 379–87.

31 Darmaun D, Mauras N. Use of stable isotopes to assess protein and amino acid metabolism in children and adolescents: a brief review. *Hormone Research*. 2005; 64(Suppl. 3): 32–7.

32 Sawka MN, Muza SR, Young, AJ. Erythrocyte volume expansion and human performance. This book, Chapter 9.

33 Nelson M, Popp H, Sharpe K, Ashenden M. Proof of homologous blood transfusion through quantification of blood group antigens. *Haematologica*. 2003; 88(11): 1284–95.

34 Voss SC, Thevis M, Schinkothe T, Schänzer W. Detection of homologous blood transfusion. *International Journal of Sports Medicine*. 2007; 28(8): 633–7.

35 Breymann, C. Erythropoietin test methods. *Baillière's Best Practice and Research Clinical Endocrinology and Metabolism*. 2000; 14(1): 135–45.

36 Lasne F. Erythropoietin doping: detection in urine. This book, Chapter 8.

37 Lasne, F, de Ceaurriz J. Recombinant erythropoietin in urine. *Nature*. 2000; 305: 635–7.

38 Lasne F. Double-blotting: a solution to the problem of non-specific binding of secondary antibodies in immunoblotting procedures. *Journal of Immunological Methods*. 2001; 253(1–2): 125–31.

39 Magnani M, Corsi D, Bianchi M, Paiardini M, Galluzzi L, Parisi A, Pigozzi F. Monitoring erythropoietin abuse in athletes. *British Journal of Haematology*. 1999; 106(1): 260–1.

40 Parisotto R, Wu M, Ashenden MJ, Emslie KR, Gore CJ, Howe C, Kazlauskas R, Sharpe K, Trout GJ, Xie M. Detection of recombinant human erythropoietin abuse in athletes utilizing markers of altered erythropoiesis. *Haematologica*. 2001; 86(2): 128–37.

41 Sharpe K, Hopkins W, Emslie KR, Howe C, Trout GJ, Kazlauskas R, Ashenden MJ, Gore CJ, Parisotto R, Hahn AG. Development of reference ranges in elite athletes for markers of altered erythropoiesis. *Haematologica*. 2002; 87(12): 1248–57.

42 Sönksen, P. Editorial. *Growth Hormone and IGF Research*. 2000; 10(3): 107–10.

43 Sönksen PH, Holt R. Growth hormones, secretogogues and related issues. This book, Chapter 10.

44 Hashimoto Y, Kamioka T, Hosaka M, Mabuchi K, Mizuchi A, Shimazaki Y, Tsunoo M, Tanaka T. Exogenous 20K growth hormone suppresses endogenous

22K growth hormone secretion in normal men. *Journal of Clinical Endocrinology and Metabolism.* 2000; 85: 601–6.

45 Longobardi S, Keay N, Ehrnborg C, Cittadini A, Rosén T, Dall R, Boroujerdi MA, Bassett EE, Healy ML, Pentecost C, Wallace JD, Powrie J, Jørgensen JO, Saccà L. The GH-2000 Study Group. Growth hormone (GH) effects on bone and collagen turnover in healthy adults and its potential as a marker of GH abuse in sports: a double blind, placebo-controlled study. *Journal of Clinical Endocrinology and Metabolism.* 2000; 85(4): 1505–12.

46 Momomura S, Hashimoto Y, Shimazaki Y, Irie M. Detection of exogenous GH administration by monitoring the ratio of 20kDa- and 22kDA-GH in serum and urine. *Endocrine Journal.* 2000; 47: 97–101.

47 Wallace JD, Cuneo RC, Lundberg PA, Rosén T, Jørgensen JO, Longobardi S, Keay N, Sacca L, Christiansen JS, Bengtsson BA, Sönksen PH. Responses of markers of bone and collagen turnover to exercise, growth hormone (GH) administration, and GH withdrawal in trained adult males. *Journal of Clinical Endocrinology and Metabolism.* 2000; 85(1): 124–33.

48 Wallace JD, Cuneo RC, Baxter R, Orskov H, Keay N, Pentecost C, Dall R, Rosén T, Jørgensen JO, Cittadini A, Longobardi S, Sacca L, Christiansen JS, Bengtsson BA, Sönksen PH. Responses of the growth hormone (GH) and insulin-like growth factor axis to exercise, GH administration, and GH withdrawal in trained adult males: a potential test for GH abuse in sport. *Journal of Clinical Endocrinology and Metabolism.* 1999; 84(10): 3591–601.

49 World Anti-Doping Agency. Gene Doping Panel. Available from http://www.wada-ama.org/en/dynamic.ch2?pageCategory.id=319 (accessed February 4, 2008).

50 Friedmann T. Gene doping. This book, Chapter 11.

51 Friedmann T. Discussion – Session 4: Enhancement 2: Potential for genetic enhancements in sports. Available from http://bioethics.gov/transcript s/jul02/session4.html (accessed February 4, 2008).

52 Recombinant DNA and Gene Transfer – Office of Biotechnology Activities. Includes *NIH guidelines for Research involving recombinant DNA molecules.* Available from http://www4.od.nih.gov/oba/Rdna.htm (accessed February 4, 2008).

53 Human gene therapy and the role of the Food and Drug Administration. Available from http://www.fda.gov/cber/infosheets/genezn.htm (accessed February 4, 2008).

54 Pipe A. Doping and its impact on the healthy athlete. This book, Chapter 13.

55 Melia P, Pipe A, Greenberg L. The use of anabolic-androgenic steroids by Canadian students. *Clinical Journal of Sport Medicine.* 1996; 6(1): 9–14.

56 Candian Centre for Ethics in Sport [homepage on the internet]. Available from www.cces.ca/ (accessed February 4, 2008).

57 Drinkwater B, Yeager KK. The female athlete triad: the inter-relatedness of disordered eating, amenorrhea, and osteoporosis. *Clinics in Sports Medicine.* 1994; 13: 405–18.

58 Hobart JA, Smucker DR. The female athlete triad (*American Family Physician.* 2000; June 1). Available from http://www.aafp.org/afp/20000601/3357.html (accessed February 4, 2008).

59 Anabolic Steroid Research Report. Available from www.steroidabuse.org (accessed February 4, 2008).

60 United States Anti-Doping Agency [homepage on the internet]. Available from http://www.usantidoping.org/ (accessed February 4, 2008).

61 Loland S, Murray TH. Editorial. The ethics of the use of technologically constructed high-altitude environments to enhance performances in sport. *Scandinavian Journal of Medicine and Science in Sports.* 2007; 17(3): 193–5.

62 Personal communication February 5, 2008 with Dr Larry D Bowers.

63 Donike M, Bärwald KR, Klostermann K, Schänzer W, Zimmermann J. Nachweis von exogenem Testosteron (Detection of exogenous testosterone). In Heck H, Hollmann W, Liesen H, Rost R, eds. *Sport: Leistung and Gesundheit.* Cologne: Deutscher Ärzte-Verlag, 1983; 293–8.

64 Special issue: Doping control. Dedicated to the memory of the late Professor Dr Manfred Donike. *Journal of Chromatography B: Analytical Technologies in the Biomedical and Life Sciences.* 1996; 687(1): 4 p preceding 1, 1–269.

Index

Page number in **bold** refer to figures, those in *italic* refer to tables.